MENTAL HEALTH AND SUBSTANCE USE DISORDERS AMONG ATHLETES

MENTAL HEALTH AND SUBSTANCE USE
DISORDERS AMONG ATHLETES

Kimberly Outlaw and Mary S. Jackson

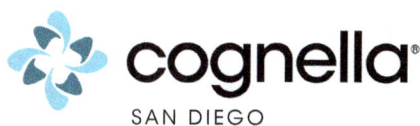

Bassim Hamadeh, CEO and Publisher
Amy Smith, Senior Project Editor
Emely Villavicencio, Senior Graphic Designer
Kylie Bartolome, Licensing Coordinator
Natalie Piccotti, Director of Marketing
Kassie Graves, Senior Vice President, Editorial
Jamie Giganti, Director of Academic Publishing

Copyright © 2024 by Cognella, Inc. All rights reserved. No part of this publication may be reprinted, reproduced, transmitted, or utilized in any form or by any electronic, mechanical, or other means, now known or hereafter invented, including pho-tocopying, microfilming, and recording, or in any information retrieval system without the written permission of Cognella, Inc. For inquiries regarding permissions, translations, foreign rights, audio rights, and any other forms of reproduction, please contact the Cognella Licensing Department at rights@cognella.com.

Trademark Notice: Product or corporate names may be trademarks or registered trademarks and are used only for identification and explanation without intent to infringe.

Cover image copyright © 2009 iStockphoto LP/RapidEye.
Cover image copyright © 2010 iStockphoto LP/garymilner.
Cover image copyright © 2016 iStockphoto LP/cmannphoto.
Cover image copyright © 2022 iStockphoto LP/ensar zengin.

Printed in the United States of America.

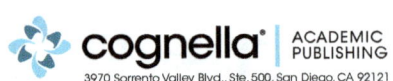

BRIEF CONTENTS

Preface		xiii
Chapter 1.	Athletes and Mental Health	1
Chapter 2.	College Athletes and Issues Related to Drug Use	9
Chapter 3.	Professional Athletes and Issues Related to Drug Use	21
Chapter 4.	Theoretical Perspectives Explaining Athletes' Behavior	27
Chapter 5.	Intersection of Race, Gender, and Nationality in Sports	51
Chapter 6.	Challenges Experienced by Athletes	57
Chapter 7.	NCAA Response to Drug Use Among Collegiate Athletes	73
Chapter 8.	The Treatment Process When Working With Athletes Who Misuse Drugs	81
Chapter 9.	Injuries as the Ultimate Gateway Drug	95
Chapter 10.	Ethics in Sports	101
Chapter 11.	Drug Use by Sport Subculture	119
Chapter 12.	Sports, Athletes, Substance Misuse: A Major Gap in Social Work Education	125
Chapter 13.	Future Challenges in Athletes Who Use Performance-Enhancing Drugs	137
Index		143

DETAILED CONTENTS

Preface   xiii

Chapter 1. Athletes and Mental Health   1

   Introduction   1
   Overview of Mental Health and Substance Abuse in Athletes   1
   Definitions and Explanation of Mental Health and Substance Use Disorders   2
   Nonprescription Drugs Used   3
   Prescription Drugs Used   5
   Prevalence of Drug Use Among Athletes   5
      Collegiate Athletes   5
      Professional Athletes   6
   Summary   6
   Discussion Questions   7
   References   7

Chapter 2. College Athletes and Issues Related to Drug Use   9

   Introduction   9
   Why Do College Athletes Use Drugs?   12
      Pain Relievers   12
      Cultural Factors   13
      Environmental Differences   14
      Victims   14
      Stress Reduction   15
      Family/Community/Fans   15
   Summary   16
   Discussion Questions   17
   References   17

Chapter 3. Professional Athletes and Issues Related to Drug Use   21

   Introduction   21
   Cultural Factors   21
      Victimization   23
      Family   23
      Community   24
      Fans   24
   Summary   25

Discussion Questions   26
References   26

Chapter 4. Theoretical Perspectives Explaining Athletes' Behavior   27

Introduction   27
Why Is There a Need to Study Theory?   28
Sociological Theories   29
- *Symbolic Interaction Theory (aka Symbolic Interactionism)*   29
- *Social Learning Theorists*   30

Psychological Theories   30
- *Psychoanalysis*   31
- *Cognitivism Theory*   32
- *Moral Stages of Development*   33
- *Operant Conditioning*   34

Biological Theories   34
- *Theories of Heredity*   35
- *Theory of Body Type*   35

Critical Theoretical Perspectives   36
- *Feminist Theory*   36
- *White Privilege*   37
- *Critical Race Theory (CRT)*   38

Models: Therapeutic Interventions   39
- *Strength-Based Perspective*   40
- *The Disease Model of Addiction*   40
- *Cognitive Behavioral Therapy (CBT)*   41
- *Motivational Interviewing*   42
- *Brief Therapy*   42
- *Moral Model*   43
- *Harm Reduction Model*   43
- *Death/Dying Model*   44

Summary   45
Discussion Questions   46
References   46

Chapter 5. Intersection of Race, Gender, and Nationality in Sports   51

Introduction   51
Historical Look at Competitive Sports   51
African Americans in Sports   52
Women in Sports   52
Racism and Sexism in Sports   52
Summary   55
Discussion Questions   55
References   56

Chapter 6. Challenges Experienced by Athletes — 57

Introduction   57
Mental Game Challenges   57
Physical Challenges   58
What About Collegiate Athletes?   59
   Balancing Athletics and Academics   60
   Balancing Social Activities With Athletic Responsibilities   60
   Balancing Athletic Success or Lack of Success   61
   Balancing Physical and Mental Health With Continued Competitiveness   61
Challenges of Trans Athletes   62
   Technological Challenges Facing Sports Industry   65
Summary   69
Discussion Questions   69
References   70

Chapter 7. NCAA Response to Drug Use Among Collegiate Athletes — 73

Introduction   73
NCAA Testing   74
Culture   75
Subculture   76
Summary   77
Discussion Questions   78
References   78

Chapter 8. The Treatment Process When Working With Athletes Who Misuse Drugs — 81

Introduction   81
Addiction Treatment for Student Athletes   83
   Addressing the Drug Abuse Among Athletes   83
Prevention, Policies, and Politics   86
Signs and Symptoms   87
Intervention Strategies   88
Federal Laws   90
   HIPAA   90
   Title 42 CFR Part 2   90
Summary   91
Discussion Questions   91
References   92

Chapter 9. Injuries as the Ultimate Gateway Drug — 95

Introduction   95
Co-Occurring Disorders Among Athletes   95
   Anxiety and Depression   96

      Eating and Exercise Disorders   96
      Substance Use Disorder   97
  Role of Injuries in Co-Occurring Disorders   97
  Counseling as a Vital Tool to Athletes   98
  Summary   99
  Discussion Questions   99
  References   100

Chapter 10. Ethics in Sports   101

  Introduction   101
  What Is Meant by Ethics?   101
  Dealing With Ethical Issues in Sports   102
      Recruitment and Punishment   103
      Academic Integrity   105
      Doping in Collegiate Sports   106
      Nanosensors   113
  Summary   115
  Discussion Questions   116
  References   116

Chapter 11. Drug Use by Sport Subculture   119

  Introduction   119
  Drugs in Sports   119
      Juiced   119
      Performance-Enhancing Drugs   120
      Regulation?   121
      Olympics   121
  Summary   122
  Discussion Questions   122
  References   122

Chapter 12. Sports, Athletes, Substance Misuse: A Major Gap in Social Work Education   125

  Introduction   125
  Doing Whatever It Takes   126
      Historical Thoughts Between Disciplines   127
      What If You Want to Counsel Athletes?   128
  Levels of Treatment   130
      The Assessment Process   130
  Gaps in Addiction Counseling   132
  Summary   133
  Discussion Questions   134
  References   135

Chapter 13. Future Challenges in Athletes Who Use Performance-Enhancing Drugs — 137

    Introduction   137
    Long-Term Effects of AAS Use   137
        Cardiovascular   137
        Fertility and Reproductive Health   138
        Psychiatric and Cognitive   138
        Other Effects   139
    Summary   139
    Discussion Questions   140
    References   140

Index   143

PREFACE

This book presents a contextualized analysis of the health issues of vulnerable populations. Population-based vulnerability is a subject of great import vis-à-vis substance abuse and mental health (SAMH). Data shows that athletes have a high SAMH vulnerability index within the global population. The competitive nature of sports exposes athletes to undue emotional and physical pressures, leading some to resort to the use of drugs such as narcotics, illegal drugs, and alcohol and suffer severe emotional, social or physical harm. There is a need to understand the mental health impacts of substance abuse among athletes. Substance abuse and mental health issues often coexist, except in isolated instances. Substance abuse inhibits personal development and causes atypical changes in personal demeanor, as well as and the development of mental issues such as trauma and depression. Besides limiting athletes' performance, substance abuse disregards the stipulated ethical code of engagement established by sporting organizations.

Substance abuse is a menace to society. In that same vein, mental health is a major cause of concern. Scholarly interests mainly seek to establish the connection between the two variables. Numerous inquiries have explored the cause-and-effect relationship between substance abuse and mental health. Others have attempted to determine the correlation between the two. Public health reports and scholarly publications have cited the prevalence of substance abuse and increased cases of addiction and depression. Yet there is still a dearth of research exploring SAMH among athletes. The book seeks to fill this research gap.

This publication is the product of 3 years of work that entailed extensive scrutiny of the available evidence, direct observation of athletes, and interrogation of key stakeholders in public health and sporting organizations—athletes, family members, and acquaintances of athletes. The nature of the discourse demanded extensive scrutiny of diverse issues to consolidate critical information required to understand SAMH among athletes in contemporary sports. The analysis did not prioritize the employment of one specific methodological approach, but instead adopted many research methods to collect both primary and secondary data. Besides scouring the internet for information from official public health institutions, the analysis examined statistical data obtained from surveys completed by various athletes. More information was obtained via interviewing consenting family, friends, colleagues, and acquaintances of athletes in various sports. In addition, qualitative data was collected from peer-reviewed publications.

The text scope covers five key areas of interest. Chapter one provides an overview of the prevalence of substance abuse in various sports ranging from cycling, athletics, and boxing to weightlifting. The analysis details the theoretical underpinnings for SAMH among athletes and discusses unique historical case studies. Chapter two examines the phenomenon of substance abuse and endeavors to present a critical analysis of key issues such as prevalence, impacts, prevention, and treatment. Chapter three explores mental health issues developed due to extensive substance abuse. In this section, the analysis relies on interviews and direct observation. Chapter four aims to establish the connection and misconceptions regarding SAMH from the perspective of athletes and offers remedial steps for averting possible addiction and trauma associated with psychological distress.

Without the many scholars who contributed to the project over the years, the background investigation and data analysis would not have been possible. We owe gratitude to the athletes, kin, acquaintances, and stakeholders who kindly agreed to participate in our studies as research subjects. The project came to fruition thanks to your efforts.

Athletes and Mental Health

INTRODUCTION

Sports are one of the great American pastimes. Many Americans revel in cheering for their favorite team or athlete. One might think that these accolades, combined with the wealth that some athletes receive, contribute to a happy and fulfilling life for athletes. The reality is, however, that many athletes struggle with mental health problems, including substance use disorders. This first chapter will shed light on this often under-discussed and under-researched area. There is much information about some athletes and how they elevated to a level of fame that captured the attention of the nation. However, there is very little information about their mental health status and use of substances as they painfully endure the victimizations of collegiate and professional athletes.

After a brief overview of this chapter and a definition of key terms, this discussion addresses drugs used by athletes, both prescription and nonprescription, and the prevalence of substance use and misuse in this population. Three discussion questions are presented at the end of the chapter, along with suggested readings and web links in the References.

OVERVIEW OF MENTAL HEALTH AND SUBSTANCE ABUSE IN ATHLETES

Athletes at all levels face great pressure to perform well and win, which can lead to mental health and substance use disorders. Effective mental health is defined throughout this text as a state of well-being with an ability to cope with stressors by the development of positive strategies to support the individual and their quest to be productive in their family, community, and nation. While most athletes experience positive mental health features, too many of them suffer from poor mental health characteristics due to the strain and stress caused by the sports profession. These athletes are the focus of this text because they suffer from poor mental health due to invisible issues that are seldom disclosed to the public. The issues remain invisible because the public only views the playing record of the athlete. Meanwhile, the stressors experienced out of the playing environment can cause the downfall of many athletes. The most reported mental health challenges among elite athletes include stress (19.6%), sleep disturbances (26.4%), anxiety and/or depression (33.6%), and alcohol misuse (18.8%) (Gouttebarge et al., 2019, p. 701). Alcohol misuse may be attributed in part to social norms among athletes and distress from transition, lack of meaningful activity, and self-treatment of pain due to injury (Gouttebarge et al., 2019, p. 705). Collegiate and professional athletes may also misuse other drugs, including marijuana, tobacco, stimulants, opioids, and anabolic steroids (Reardon & Creado, 2014, p. 96).

Drugs usage by professional or collegiate sports players may result in addiction to illegal substances and psychiatric disorders. Performance enhancement drugs also increase the need for addiction specialists, of which there is a shortage in the sports domain. Still, in the last few decades, performance enhancing drugs or PEDs have become more prevalent problems.

DEFINITIONS AND EXPLANATION OF MENTAL HEALTH AND SUBSTANCE USE DISORDERS

Mental health refers to one's "emotional, psychological, and social well-being" (U.S. Department of Health and Human Services, 2020). Several factors contribute to mental health, including biological factors such as genetics or neurochemistry, life experiences such as trauma or abuse, and a family history of psychological disorders. The *Diagnostic and Statistical Manual of Mental Disorders* (DSM-5) provides guidelines for labeling mental disorders and is considered the universal tool used by health care professionals when providing treatment for clients with mental health issues. Twenty mental health disorders are delineated by the DSM-5 (APA, 2013), and each disorder is associated with different symptoms and outcomes. Some warning signs common to more than one disorder include changes in appetite, reduced energy levels, social withdrawal, apathy, feelings of hopelessness, mood swings, anxiety, thoughts of self-harm, visual or auditory hallucinations, and the inability to carry out tasks of daily living, such as those associated with work or school (U.S. Department of Health and Human Services, 2020).

Substance use disorder is one category of mental health disorder. While each type of substance may be identified as a specific disorder, such as alcohol use disorder or opioid use disorder, the criteria for each of these is generally the same. The DSM-5 defines a substance use disorder as "a problematic pattern of substance use leading to clinically significant impairment or distress, as manifested by at least two of the following symptoms occurring within a 12-month period" (Saunders, 2017, p. 232):

- craving or strong desire to use the substance
- unsuccessfully attempting to cut back on use
- using the substance more often or in greater amounts than intended
- suffering inability to fulfill responsibilities at work, school, or home
- spending significant amounts of time obtaining or using the substance
- continuing to use the substance despite the problems it causes
- building tolerance to the substance
- experiencing withdrawal symptoms

- continuing to use the substance despite associated physical or psychological problems
- using the substance in dangerous situations
- giving up important activities due to the substance use (Saunders, 2017, p. 232)

These criteria apply to three different categories of drugs, as well as other or unknown substances and behavioral addictions, including gambling and internet gambling. The class of drugs categorized as central nervous system (CNS) depressants includes alcohol, marijuana, inhalants, opioids, sedatives, hypnotics, and anxiolytics. The class of drugs categorized as CNS stimulants includes tobacco, caffeine, and stimulants. Drugs belonging to the hallucinogen/empathogen/dissociative category include all types of hallucinogens (Saunders, 2017, p. 229).

NONPRESCRIPTION DRUGS USED

Athletes at all levels may use drugs for a variety of reasons. They may use them to cope with the stress of being an athlete, including overcoming the pressure to perform. In addition, they may use drugs to relieve pain or treat injuries or to cope with the stress and change associated with retirement from their sport (Reardon & Creado, 2014, p. 95). Substance abuse seems to be a double-edged analgesic for some athletes. While athletes may receive comprehensive treatment for physical conditions, they are less likely to receive help for mental health conditions, due in part to the stigma associated with mental illness. As a result, untreated mental illness can result in substance abuse, which can lead to substance use disorder. Conversely, substance abuse can lead to other forms of mental illness (Reardon & Creado, 2014, p. 96).

Many athletes at all levels use and abuse a wide variety of drugs—tobacco, alcohol, marijuana, anabolic steroids, opioids, and stimulants (Reardon & Creado, 2014, p. 96). Of these, the use of performance-enhancing drugs is particularly relevant, and the primary type of performance-enhancing drug is anabolic steroids. These drugs cannot be legally obtained in the United States without a prescription and are banned in professional sports by the World Anti-Doping Agency (WADA) (Reardon & Creado, 2014, p. 97; University of Michigan Health, 2019).

While anabolic steroids can be prescribed, they are included in this section because some athletes may obtain them illegally. In addition, other nonprescription substances can serve to enhance performance. The category of performance-enhancing drugs includes androgens, growth hormones and growth factors, stimulants, nutritional supplements, and diuretics (Rearson & Creado, 2014, p. 98).

Androgens, also known as anabolic steroids, are hormones used to increase testosterone in males. Increased testosterone promotes the development of muscle mass and strength (Reardon & Creado, 2014, p. 98). Examples of anabolic steroids used to promote increased testosterone include fluoxymesterone and nandrolone. When obtained illegally, they are typically taken at doses up to 100 times higher than what a physician would prescribe for legal uses (University of Michigan Health, 2019). The term *stacking* refers to taking more than one anabolic steroid at a time. The term *pyramiding* refers to cycling between no drug and a high dose of the drug over several weeks or months (University of Michigan Health, 2019). While these drugs may be effective at building muscle, there are significant drawbacks in taking them. In men, anabolic steroids can lead to reduced sperm counts, reduced testicle size, sterility, and enlarged breasts. Women who take these drugs may experience increased body hair, decreased breast size, and a deepened voice. Both and woman may experience rage, aggression, violence, mania, delusions, and substance use disorder. In addition, these drugs increase the risk of hypertension, heart attack, stroke, high cholesterol, liver disease, acne, and skin infections (University of Michigan Health, 2019).

A second type of performance-enhancing drug is growth hormones/growth factors. Recombinant growth hormone can increase muscle mass and decrease fat mass, as well as improve sprinting capacity. Growth factors such as insulin-like growth factor (IGF-1) and insulin may have effects similar to that of growth hormone, but these have not been extensively studied in athletes (Reardon & Creado, 2014, p. 98). Guha et al. (2013) noted that, at least at the time of publication, there were no confirmed cases of IGIF-1 misuse among athletes. However, the drug was popular with amateur bodybuilders as evidenced by extensive discussion in online forums, including how to use it alone or in combination with growth hormone. Reported advantages included increased muscle size and strength, increased energy and endurance, improved immunity, and increased bone density (p. 9670). At least two pharmaceutical companies manufacture IGF-1 under the names Increlex and iPlex (Guha et al., 2013, p. 9670).

Stimulants may also enhance performance among athletes. This class of drugs includes amphetamine, D-methamphetamine, methylphenidate, ephedrine, pseudoephedrine, caffeine, and cocaine among others. These types of drugs improve endurance, anaerobic performance, reaction time, and alertness, while decreasing fatigue (Reardon & Creado, 2014, p. 99). All but caffeine is banned by the WADA. Athletes may obtain caffeine in a number of ways, including through energy drinks that may contain up to 500 mg caffeine per can or bottle. While many drinks or foods containing caffeine may contain too little to impact athletic performance, Ribeiro et al. (2017) reported that a dose of 6 mg/kg body weight was effective at improving time trial performance. However, the authors noted that caffeine at this and other doses did not impact muscle power or endurance (p. 288).

Like caffeine, nutritional supplements are not banned by WADA. This category of performance enhancers includes vitamins, minerals, herbs, and extracts. The specific benefit varies according to the supplement.

Creatine is a popular supplement and one that is not banned by the WADA. This substance increased power output and lean body mass (Reardon & Creado, 2014, p. 99). While short-term use of this supplement is considered safe, few studies have investigated the long-term effects. Isolated cases of liver damage exist, however these cases typically involved excessive or inappropriate use of creatine (Butts, Jacobs, & Silvis, 2018, p. 33).

A final category of performance enhancing substances is diuretics. Diuretics are used to induce rapid weight loss through water loss, often in combat sports such as wrestling, boxing, or karate, where an athlete's weight may determine his competitor (Franchini et al., 2012, p. 1). Data linking the use of diuretics with success in these sports is conflicting. However, notable psychological and physiological effects exist from using diuretics to induce weight loss before a competition. Athletes may experience decreased short-term memory, concentration, and self-esteem, as well as increased depression, confusion, rage, and fatigue (Franchini et al., 2012, p. 3). Physiological effects include decreased aerobic and anaerobic performance, dehydration, decreased plasma volume, and increased heart rate (Franchini et al., 2012, p. 4).

PRESCRIPTION DRUGS USED

In addition to illegally obtained substances and nutritional supplements, some athletes may take prescription medications obtained from a licensed physician. One can imagine that opioids are likely to be a common drug prescribed for some athletes, such as football players who sustain frequent injuries. Cottler et al. (2011) surveyed 644 retired professional football players regarding opioid use. Almost one-half of the sample reported having at least one concussion and/or three or more injuries while playing (Cottler et al., 2011, p. 5), and 52% of the sample reported using opioids during their football career. Only 37% of these individuals obtained them legally from a physician, and 71% of these admitted to abusing opioids during their career. These individuals were 3.2-fold more likely to continue misusing the drugs after retirement compared with players who used them as directed (Cottler et al., 2011, p. 5).

Some college athletes also misuse prescription stimulants. This class of drugs, which can enhance performance, includes Adderall, Ritalin, and Concerta. Gallucci and Martin (2015) reported that 7.5% of college athletes reported misusing prescription stimulant medications in the past year. More than half of these individuals obtained the medication from another person rather than misusing their own prescription (p. 47). Reasons for misuse included longer study time, to improved mental focus, and better concentration in class (p. 48). These are not surprising reasons, given the high demand placed upon collegiate athletes to succeed, not only on the field but also in the classroom.

PREVALENCE OF DRUG USE AMONG ATHLETES

Collegiate Athletes

The prevalence of drug use among college athletes varies according to the specific drug. In a review of the literature, Reardon and Creado (2014) reported that the prevalence of alcohol use within this group ranged from 75% to 93% among male athletes and 71% to 93% among female athletes (p. 96). Among collegiate athletes, 28% report using marijuana in the preceding year, and 3% report using stimulants (p. 96). College athletes also use smokeless tobacco, the prevalence of which may vary by sport. During the preceding year, 23% of college athletes in general report using this substance, compared with up to 50% of collegiate baseball players (p. 96). Collegiate and even high school athletes use anabolic steroids, although at a much lower frequency than other drugs. According to Reardon and Creado (2014), between 0.7% and 6.6% of high school athletes use anabolic steroids, as do 0.2% to 5% of male collegiate athletes and up to 1.6% of female collegiate athletes (p. 96).

Many athletes may use more than one substance. The use of more than one substance at a time, or polysubstance use, differs according to athlete characteristics. According to Orsini et al. (2018) differences exist with regard to gender, race, and athletic division. In this study of over 3,200 collegiate athletes, the authors reported that a greater percentage of men than women used both alcohol and tobacco, at 13.4% and 4.1%, respectively (p. 192). Of all combinations of substances addressed by the authors, which included various combinations of alcohol, tobacco, marijuana, and prescription drugs, alcohol and tobacco was the most prevalent combination. The use of this combination was far more prevalent among American Indian or Alaskan Natives than any other race, at 17.6% of athletes surveyed. In fact, drug use among athletes in this cultural group was more prevalent than in any other cultural group in the survey (Orsini et al., 2018, p. 192). While athletes in all three divisions used alcohol with tobacco at about the same rate, ranging from 7.6% to 9.8%, Division III athletes used alcohol and marijuana at a rate five-fold higher than Division I athletes. In general, polysubstance abuse is more prevalent among Division III athletes than among athletes in the other two divisions (Orsini et al., 2018, p. 192).

It is important to note that the articles cited in this section, including Reardon and Creado (2014) and Orsini et al. (2018) used self-report data. In other words, the athletes themselves reported their own use of drugs. Although assurances of anonymity and confidentiality may help to promote honesty, self-report data is associated with biases. Given that drug and alcohol use is a sensitive subject with potentially serious repercussions, athletes may tend to underreport their usage due to fear of disclosure (Druckman et al., 2015, p. 370). These concerns are not unwarranted. The National Collegiate Athletics Association (NCAA) bans substances such as anabolic steroids, stimulants, illicit drugs, and large amounts of caffeine. Alcohol is not necessarily banned, but the NCAA warns athletes not to overuse this substance. Athletes who use these substances may be banned from participation in sports (Druckman et al., 2015, p. 371). In addition, drug use is typically a socially undesirable behavior, and individuals may underreport their use based on the need for social acceptance (Druckman et al., 2015, p. 370). The key point is that studies relying on self-report data may underreport actual drug use prevalence.

Professional Athletes

In some cases, the prevalence of drug use among professional athletes is higher than that of collegiate athletes. For example, while up to 5% of collegiate athletes use anabolic steroids, about 9% of professional football players and 67% of competitive power lifters use these drugs (Reardon & Creado, 2014, p. 96). Another type of performance enhancement is blood doping, which refers to the use of blood transfusions or drugs to increase red blood cells and oxygen capacity. An average of 14% of elite track and field athletes across the world engage in this practice (Sottas et al., 2011, p. 766). In addition, up to 40% and up to 30% of professional baseball and football players, respectively, use smokeless tobacco, compared with 23% of all collegiate athletes (Reardon & Creado, 2014, p. 96). With respect to opiates, 52% of professional athletes report using this drug type at some point in their careers, and 71% of these individuals report misusing the drug (Reardon & Creado, 2014, p. 96).

SUMMARY

Athletes at all levels can face great pressure to perform and succeed. While many athletes cope well with these pressures, a notable number develop mental health issues or substance use disorders. The types of drugs used by collegiate and professional athletes include performance-enhancing drugs such as anabolic steroids, growth hormones, stimulants, nutritional supplements, and diuretics, as well as other drugs like opioids to relieve pain from injury and prescription stimulants to maintain concentration in class. In addition, substances such as tobacco, alcohol, and marijuana are also used and misused by some athletes. Among collegiate athletes, the most frequently used substances are alcohol and marijuana, and a number of athletes use more than one drug. Native American and Native Alaskan athletes are particularly susceptible to drug use, with higher prevalence than athletes of other races. In the professional realm, athletes tend to use anabolic steroids and tobacco more frequently than college athletes. In addition, almost half of professional football players used opioids during their careers to treat injury-related pain, and almost three-quarters of these players misused the drug. Clearly, substance use and abuse is a significant concern among collegiate and professional athletes. These individuals face unique challenges and pressures not typically faced by the general population. Effective substance use treatments and prevention programs are paramount for this population.

DISCUSSION QUESTIONS

1. Do you recall professional or collegiate athletes that have struggled publicly with drug or alcohol abuse? How did it affect their performance?
2. What steps do you think coaches can take to help prevent substance use and abuse among athletes?
3. What factors might prevent a collegiate or professional athlete from seeking treatment for mental health issues?

REFERENCES

American Psychiatric Association. (2013). *Diagnostic and statistical manual of mental disorders* (5th ed.).

Butts, J., Jacobs, B., & Silvis, M. (2018). Creatine use in sports. *Sports Health, 10*(1), 31–34.

Cottler, L. B., Ben Abdallah, A., Cummings, S. M., Barr, J., Banks, R., & Forchheimer, R. (2011). Injury, pain, and prescription opioid use among former National Football League (NFL) players. *Drug and Alcohol Dependence, 116*(1–3), 188–194. https://doi.org/10.1016/j.drugalcdep.2010.12.003

Druckman, J. N., Gilli, M., Klar, S., & Robison, J. (2015). Measuring drug and alcohol use among college student-athletes. *Social Science Quarterly, 96*(2), 369–380.

Franchini, E., Brito, C. J., & Artioli, G. G. (2012). Weight loss in combat sports: Physiological, psychological and performance effects. *Journal of the International Society of Sports Nutrition, 9*(1), 1–6.

Gallucci, A. R., & Martin, R. J. (2015). Misuse of prescription stimulant medication in a sample of college students: Examining differences between varsity athletes and non-athletes. *Addictive Behaviors, 51*, 44–50.

Gouttebarge, V., Castaldelli-Maia, J. M., Gorczynski, P., Hainline, B., Hitchcock, M. E., Kerkhoffs, G. M., … & Reardon, C. L. (2019). Occurrence of mental health symptoms and disorders in current and former elite athletes: A systematic review and meta-analysis. *British Journal of Sports Medicine, 53*(11), 700–706.

Guha, N., Cowan, D. A., Sönksen, P. H., & Holt, R. I. (2013). Insulin-like growth factor-I (IGF-I) misuse in athletes and potential methods for detection. *Analytical and Bioanalytical Chemistry, 405*(30), 9669–9683.

Orsini, M. M., Milroy, J. J., Wyrick, D. L., & Sanders, L. (2018). Polysubstance use among first-year NCAA college student-athletes. *Journal of Child & Adolescent Substance Abuse, 27*(3), 189–195.

Reardon, C. L., & Creado, S. (2014). Drug abuse in athletes. *Substance Abuse and Rehabilitation, 5,* 95–105. https://doi.org/10.2147/SAR.S53784

Ribeiro, B. G., Morales, A. P., Sampaio-Jorge, F., de Souza Tinoco, F., Matos, A. A., & Leite, T. C. (2017). Acute effects of caffeine intake on athletic performance: A systematic review and meta-analysis. *Revista Chilena de Nutrición, 44*(3), 283–291.

Saunders, J. B. (2017). Substance use and addictive disorders in DSM-5 and ICD 10 and the draft ICD 11. *Current Opinion in Psychiatry, 30*(4), 227–237.

Sottas, P. E., Robinson, N., Fischetto, G., Dollé, G., Alonso, J. M., & Saugy, M. (2011). Prevalence of blood doping in samples collected from elite track and field athletes. *Clinical Chemistry, 57*(5), 762–769.

University of Michigan Health. (2019). Anabolic steroids: What are anabolic steroids? https://www.uofmhealth.org/health-library/za1277#:~:text=In%20the%20United%20States%2C%20you,made%20by%20the%20human%20body

U.S. Department of Health and Human Services. (2020). What is mental health? https://www.mentalhealth.gov/basics/what-is-mental-health

College Athletes and Issues Related to Drug Use

INTRODUCTION

Drugs have existed in civilization as long as human life has existed. Drugs are mind-altering substances that impact individuals based on quantity (amount taken) and potency (ingredients). In the United States, drugs are categorized into five schedules, by the Drug Enforcement Administration (DEA), based on medicinal use and dependency qualities. The DEA has the responsibility for categorizing drugs into their specific schedules under the Controlled Substances Act (CSA) of 1970, which was signed into law by former president Nixon. The CSA is the first unified framework for the regulation of federally controlled substances (Lampe, 2021). The CSA grants authority to the DEA along with Food and Drug Administration (FDA) to decide which substances are medically useful (DEA, 2021). The feature that determines which schedule of category a drug is placed into is based not only on medical usefulness but also on the rate of abuse of the drug. For example, schedule I drugs can cause a high rate of abuse resulting in psychological and physical dependence (e.g., heroin) and schedule V drugs have a low potential for abuse (e.g., codeine less than 200 milligrams). The following controlled substances chart is relevant to view and to keep in mind while reading this chapter.

TABLE 2.1 Controlled Substances Chart

Schedule I Drugs	Heroin, lysergic acid diethylamide (LSD), marijuana (cannabis), 3,4-methylenedioxymethamphetamine (ecstasy), methaqualone, bath salts, and peyote
Schedule II Drugs	Combination products with less than 15 milligrams of hydrocodone per dosage unit (Vicodin), cocaine, morphine, methamphetamine, methadone, hydromorphone (Dilaudid), meperidine (Demerol), oxycodone (OxyContin), fentanyl, Dexedrine, Adderall, and Ritalin
Schedule III Drugs	Products containing less than 90 milligrams of codeine per dosage unit (Tylenol with codeine), ketamine, anabolic steroids, testosterone, Vicodin, Suboxone
Schedule IV Drugs	Xanax, Soma, Darvon, Darvocet, Valium, Ativan, Talwin, Ambien, Tramadol
Schedule V Drugs	Cough preparations with less than 200 milligrams of codeine or per 100 milliliters (Robitussin AC), Lomotil, Motofen, Lyrica, Parepectolin

Source: United States Drug Enforcement Administration. DEA.gov is an official site of the U.S. Department of Justice. https://www.dea.gov/drug-scheduling

There are some issues related to the classification system, and a major debate continues surrounding the classification of marijuana as a schedule I drug. The argument has been that marijuana is not as dangerous as heroin and therefore should not receive the same harsh criminal sanctions (Lopez, 2016). However, the DEA continues to classify marijuana as a schedule I drug because there is not enough scientific evidence to suggest the medicinal value. Thus, marijuana remains on the schedule I category list of high-risk potentially dangerous drugs and yet can be found on every college and university campus in the United States.

The marijuana issue places America in another dilemma with the federal government agency (DEA) classifying it as a schedule I drug, while since 1996 federally funding marijuana growers in the United States. Hawryluk (2019) reports that after 20 years, legal marijuana growers supported by the federal government have the best marijuana products in the world. However, because it is still an illegal product (federally illegal even if legal in some states) it cannot be sold commercially. Even the largest cannabis hybrid greenhouse in Nevada cannot export its marijuana product due to the federal laws. Thus, Canada, which legalized marijuana in 2018, became the world's leading marijuana export (Hawryluk, 2019). Although the argument is that there is time for America to "catch up," Americans are extremely competitive and it is likely that this Canadian marijuana business will impact the stock market, in turn influencing the U.S. government to reclassify marijuana. Many governmental decisions are made on the basis of the stock market. The reclassification of marijuana is no different. As of December 2020, the trend can be seen in the shift of 15 states and the District of Columbia passing laws approving recreational and medical marijuana use and 33 states legalizing medicinal marijuana use and the use of cannabidiol (CBD) (Lampe, 2021). With the legalization of marijuana, it is important to be prepared for the impact not only on the health care system, but the world of sports and especially college athletes.

The debate regarding whether there are harmful effects to recreational marijuana use continues. Memedovich et al. (2018) suggest that recreational marijuana use has harmful effects, citing more than 60 journal articles to support the negative effects. They revealed that evidence of harm was reported in 62 reviews of mental health disorders, pregnancy outcomes, testicular cancer, cognitive outcomes, and brain changes. Karst (2018) considers both positive and negative effects of marijuana use (asthenia, balance problems, disorientation, gastrointestinal effects, euphoria, somnolence, dry mouth, fatigue, hallucinations, paranoia, and agitation as the most commonly reported effects). She further points out that studies reviewing long-term effects of marijuana use have revealed negative effects associated with psychotic disorders and worsening symptoms of PTSD. She strongly encourages the need for further research due to the inconsistencies of research studies regarding the harmful effects and due to the lack of quality standards and regulations by FDA for medical marijuana.

The counterargument for the use or legalization of marijuana is based on the foundation that cannabis sativa is a natural phytomedicine that has been used in folk medicine for thousands of years to treat sleep problems (insomnia, induce sleep, soporific); arthritis and pain (gout, rheumatism, and arthritic pain); gynecological disorders (dysmenorrhea, menorrhagia, expedite delivery); sexual problems (erectile dysfunction, sex stimulation, low libido, pleasant sensation); gastrointestinal problems (diarrhea, dyspepsia, strangulated hernia, poor digestion, dysentery); neuropsychiatric and CNS (paralysis, psychosis, insanity); infections and respiratory problems (tetanus, wound, tuberculosis, cough, asthma);

cancer; and other ailments including hypertension, headache, itch, lack of bile secretion, abortifacient, dandruff, fever, and urinary problems (Shahriar et al., 2021). The authors conclude there is a need for further studies to assist with the formulation of therapeutic guidelines in preparation for future emerging challenges.

Regardless of the discussion at large, the NCAA has taken a different passion on their previous ban on marijuana use among college athletes. In the past, if an athlete tests positive for marijuana use in a drug test, the athlete would be declared ineligible for future competition and withheld from 50% of their competition in all of their competitive sports (NCAA, 2017b). However, there has been a change in the NCAA's position on marijuana use among college athletes. The recent change became effective February 23, 2022, which increases the acceptable THC levels from 35 nanograms per milliliter to 150 nanograms per milliliter (Golembeski, 2022). This implies that the NCAA has changed its position from zero tolerance to a percentage level that will be acceptable without penalty to the athlete (loss of eligibility). This policy change could have occurred based on U.S. public opinion regarding marijuana and a similar position taken by the World Anti-Doping Agency with the thinking that marijuana does not impede the athlete's performance (Golembeski, 2022).

Marijuana has been discussed extensively here because it is one of the primary drugs of choice among college athletes. The other two drugs of choice among college athletes are alcohol and tobacco. Lopez (2016) suggests that the two recreational drugs—alcohol and tobacco—were not included on the CSA schedule in 1970 because they received specific exemption from scheduling. Based on congressional perspectives, the term *substance* does not include distilled spirits, wine, malt beverages, or tobacco. The congressional thinking is that those terms are defined or used in subtitle E of the Internal Revenue Code of 1986. Therefore, Congress made the decision to exempt alcohol and tobacco from CSA (SAMHSA, 2016). However, congress is also receiving pressure under the marijuana backdrop to revisit the issue of alcohol and tobacco for inclusion on CSA.

The use of illicit drugs and alcohol among college students is a phenomenon that continues in American society with no institution of higher education exempt from the situation. This is inclusive of public and private schools, ivy league schools, and rural and urban programs. The National Collegiate Athletic Association (NCAA) reports that there are 480,000 student athletes, 19,300 teams, 1,100 member schools, and 3 divisions (NCAA, 2017a). Many of these students participate in drug use, including alcohol, tobacco, marijuana, and illicit drugs.

It should be noted, however, that illicit drug and alcohol use for many college students does not begin on the college campus. Often the use started in high school and was simply exacerbated with college entrance. The gateway hypothesis (Choo et al., 2008) suggests that the use of illicit drugs such as alcohol and tobacco begins in middle and high school, which serves as a pathway for continuing to use drugs and adding other drugs during higher education (Barry et al., 2016; Kirby & Barry, 2012). Full-time college students are twice as likely to use illicit drugs and alcohol as individuals who do not attend college (Addiction Center, 2021). They comprise the largest group of drug abusers in the nation (ages 18–22), with 54.9% reporting drinking in the previous month—higher by 10% than non-college students (Moore & Abbe, 2021). College athletes are subgroups within colleges and universities that participate in the consumption of drugs and alcohol.

WHY DO COLLEGE ATHLETES USE DRUGS?

College students typically use drugs to socialize and belong (experiencing peer pressure), to ease stress over grades (struggling with working and taking classes within a specific time frame), and to feel the excitement of being away from home (making decisions based on limited experience and guidance). These factors can push them into drug use/abuse. However, athletes have different stressors that move them into the drug-taking arena.

From an outsider perspective, an athlete may seem to have everything. Individuals will remark, "They have everything; why are they using drugs?" What is frequently missing from the equation is the fact that the athlete does not really have everything. The athlete is just like every other college student, with the difference being that the athlete is frequently in the spotlight. This spotlight brings additional pressures when winning becomes the focus. The pressures surrounding the need to win are so paramount that the athlete is willing to succumb to factors such as approved victimization, frustrations, self-doubt, and pain, which other college students may never experience. Therefore, many college athletes are driven to drugs to relieve pain (physical and psychological), as a coping strategy (against victimization), for stress reduction (academic performance/financial issues), and to alleviate the frustrations and fear of being cut from the team.

Pain Relievers

Imagine moving away from home for the first time and living with strangers or non-relatives. That can be rather scary. But include in that scenario the notion of a star athlete who has signed an agreement with a major school of higher education to perform at the highest level in a college sport. In high school the task may have been easy where everyone grew up together from the same neighborhood. Parents knew each other and supported each other at games and arranged carpools around game celebrations. Then comes college, where a signature on a piece of paper suggests that you must perform well or become eliminated and sent home. In college there are diverse groups with everyone making performance decisions. Other athletes appear to be bigger and better and there is a need to prove an outstanding performance. In addition, there is the need to attend classes that are large with unfamiliar professors who do not appear to recognize the name or the sport. The lecture information appears to be foreign, and yet there is the expectation that classroom attendance is necessary (or is it?). Rigorous training schedules and many physical hits in practice by other teammates who would like to take the playing position becomes a lonely time of continuous self-doubt, pain, and fear.

Meanwhile, a happy ambitious face must be displayed to everyone. There is no one to discuss these feelings with because, although a psychological counseling center is located on the main campus, it is taboo for an athlete striving to make good on a contractual agreement to be viewed as "having mental problems." Discussions are limited with the family because the family is so proud—pain from injury or aloneness is often not discussed. When an athlete is not performing well, they may skip times with the family to elude discussions about college life and sports. And, even though team comradery is emphasized in the locker room, few college athletes discuss feelings of loneliness with teammates for fear that they may be perceived differently or that the teammate may reveal the information to the coach. Therefore, the athlete may turn to illegal drugs or overuse prescription drugs to relieve the pain. Villa

(2019) states that college athletes will suffer through pain, which she terms the "culture of pain," and painful events to play the sport, putting competition above everything else.

Athletes injured on the field may be prescribed Oxycontin, which can lead to heroin use. Low cost and easy access on the internet or on the street can be extremely dangerous because heroin can be laced with fentanyl. The athlete who gravitates to using heroin is quickly released to return home, which then becomes a breeding ground for intensification of pain relievers, unless there are treatment interventions.

According to the NCAA, depression and anxiety are the most commonly reported psychological issues among student athletes (Hainline et al., n.d.). Some student athletes may use alcohol to deal with depression because, after all, the NCAA does not consider alcohol a rejectable drug (unless it becomes a disease). It is interesting that, while the NCAA started drug testing in 1986 and included in 2003 testing for caffeine concentration (15 micrograms per milliliter in the body as restrictive) (Chang, 2018), alcohol screening is not included. The drug classes banned by NCAA are stimulants, anabolic agents, diuretics and other masking agents, narcotics, cannabinoids, peptide hormones, growth factors, related substances, and mimetics, hormone and metabolic modulators (anti-estrogens), and beta-2 agonists. Alcohol and beta blockers are banned for rifle use only (NCAA, 2021). Yet, alcohol is the most commonly used substance among college students and athletes (Skidmore et al., 2016).

Cultural Factors

Culture plays a central role in substance use/abuse among college athletes. *Culture* is used in the context of an integrated set of goals, values, beliefs, and attitudes that are mutually experienced in a shared society or within particular groups. Within societal cultures are subcultures, and college athletes are a subculture. The Chicago School used a framework to define subculture within a deviance contextual foundation (Williams, 2007), suggesting that social and environmental factors affect the choices and performances made by individuals as they function in their subgroup. Although college athletes come together from different societal experiences, when they come together on the college campus as college athletes, they become a team with the indoctrination from coaches that they must perform well in order to remain members of the team. The athletes may discover that although the cultural (societal) and subcultural (team) expectations are similar (they must perform well), the treatment is different, and these differences can cause many negative challenges for them. They become isolated from the general college population, yet they are expected to interact (to a degree) with the general college population at social events. Athletes are housed in special units and their needs are taken care of by the athletic department, which is generally away from other campus units. Special staff are assigned to the athletic department (medical doctors, tutors, special assistants, and mentors). Unfortunately, many of these special staff accommodations are also focused on the coach's goal (winning games at all costs). Academic schedules are controlled by the athletic department with advisors developing schedules to accommodate the best workout and practice times. Sometimes advisors select classes that are deemed "easy," without regard for the athlete's future goals. They may create a schedule where required general classes may be "skipped" or assign tutors to "work" on their class assignments or sign the class attendance sheet for the athlete who needs to report to training during the same time as the scheduled class. Athletic departments are the most equipped departments on campuses and they receive the highest amount of funding, yet they continue to be allowed to function in isolation without close monitoring from university administrators as long as they produce winning seasons. These young athletes seldom understand the dual roles, but they experience the feelings of confusion, and many turn to alcohol as a means of coping. Athletes, participants in Greek organizations, sexual minorities, those who suffer from depression and anxiety, and White males seem to be at particular risk for substance abuse during college (Skidmore et al., 2016).

Environmental Differences

The college campus can be a frightening experience for incoming students who are away from home for the first time and living without the protection of their parents. It can also be frightening for athletes. Although they may have reported to campus months ahead of other students, their acculturation process differs because they must not only incorporate the values, beliefs, and customs of the team, but also the values, beliefs, and customs of the college or university when all students are on campus. They discover differences within the two cultures that cause stress. For example, the team rules, policies, and routines (e.g., training) are strenuous and demanding. However, due to their status on campus as college athletes, they are privileged in many instances: They are invited to parties, they are allowed special progress reports, they receive special college or university excused absences from class, and they have special study areas within the athletic department. This "special" treatment deviates from the team treatment, especially if they do not perform well on the field or court. Therefore, there is the constant struggle among college athletes to remember which demeanor to portray, depending on the environment.

For example, coaches dissuade athletes from engaging in using illegal drugs and alcohol. However, when athletes attend parties such as Greek parties, this behavior is welcomed and encouraged. Weaver (2020) and Salas-Wright, Vaughn, and Gonzalez (2016) suggest that participation in Greek life is associated with drug use (smoking, marijuana use, and alcohol). The use of drugs can lower the athlete's performance. Even with this knowledge the motivation is extremely high among college athletes to participate in Greek life as a means to what they may consider a balance between torture (harsh training under coaches) and pleasure (partying). However, many athletes are not physically and mentally able to handle the stress of attempting to balance the two worlds, and they do not discuss their conflicting feelings. Thus, they become victims to their personal imposed nightmares, which push them further into drinking and drugging in an effort to feel better. They do not understand that the temporary feeling of pleasure is simply an escape that will cause them greater harm in the future.

Victims

Coaches are considered surrogate parental figures to college athletes. Away from home regardless of what the home situation was at the time, these athletes are young, ambitious, and vulnerable. The coaches become the substitute enforcer. The concept of substitute enforcer is used as opposed to substitute parent because many parents would not victimize their children for a game win. However, to coaches the game win is the most important component when discussing college athletes. Their future contractual services to the college depend on the number of games won. This is not to imply that coaches do not care about their players, but the implication here is that college athletics is a business and the coaches are simply business partners with the college. It is clearly understood that the coaches must win games in order to remain at the college. Therefore, their goal is to produce winning teams at whatever the costs to the players. Players are expendable and expected to become permissive victims under the coach's tutelage. Players are told when to sleep, when to eat, when to train, when to when to see their parents, and not to violate the coach's rules (whatever the rules are).

According to a 2015 NCAA drug survey of 20,000 athletes, 24% of college athletes reported that their coach knew they were taking drugs (steroids). The survey documented, "21 percent say their coach, athletic trainer, or team physician supplies the drugs." As a result of the 2015 survey results the NCAA introduced a new drug testing policy where players would be randomly tested for drugs. However, there is no mention or any indication that there are policies to deter coaches and other staff from providing drugs to players (NCAA, 2017b). This is a major area of concern as players continue to become victimized in the organizational scheme with no enforcements or sanctions for coaches or team staff who encourage or look the other way to avoid assisting a player who experiences psychological issues. The goal is to ensure that the player's physical body is in shape to play the next game.

Stress Reduction

College athletes experience a great deal of stress that often goes unnoticed due to the false façade of the glory of winning the game and "teammate ship" (it is all about the team). The image is depicted of the happy-go-lucky athlete who is adored by everyone on and off campus (within the television viewing audience), but behind that fake happiness, is a cloud of fear, anger, and uncertainty—the fear of not measuring up to the coach's and the team's expectations in the sports arena. There is always another player seeking the same playing position and the constant focus is on not become injured and scoring as many points as possible. If an injury should occur, the fear intensifies as eligibility becomes a haunting concern. Anger emerges within the player as the search for answers becomes a relentless search ending with limited positive outcomes. This anger forces players to become constant reminders of their vulnerabilities. The strength and power that was displayed on the playing field is no longer visible as a weakened ego emerges with a need for support. When the athlete cannot obtain positive support, drugs become a source and a means for depressing anger and thoughts of future failures.

Family/Community/Fans

Financial burdens and academic performance are relevant in this discussion about stress reduction because many college athletes obtain sports scholarships and would otherwise have no other means to enroll in a college or university. Many of them have been ill prepared in high school to perform well in college. They know and understand their level of functioning academically is a matter of self-mentoring, locating a mentor to assist with academic assignments. Or they can sit in the back of the room as a group of athletes who are attempting to achieve their goals. These athletes understand that they must remain in school, and yet it becomes a major struggle for many of them when they are ill prepared and when there are limited efforts on the part of the college or university to prepare them academically. Although higher institutions proclaim in their mission statements the goal to provide quality education for their students, too few will provide the time and effort to ensure that athletes leave with a quality education. Many may not graduate, and some elite athletes may graduate but be unable to read or write simple sentences.

Some families are unable to advocate for their children because they are unaware of how to navigate within the higher education system. They may not have been able to navigate in the high school system to demand quality academic standards for their child. The joy of having their child in college as a potential professional player (long-term goal) is often the aim for many families who have a child entering the higher education arena. For many of these parents, the potential of earning millions of dollars in the future outweighs gaining quality education. While some academicians and parents may negatively criticize athletes who leave college for the pros without earning their degree, it is relevant to remember that their long-term goal (to enter professional sports) outweighs education when participation in the professional sport can remove a family from living in poverty.

Communities or neighborhoods are generally supportive of the college-bound athlete and provide kudos when they are successful. However, many families of athletes receive minimal community support and many struggle with financial challenges during the time that the student is in college. Although the athlete is receiving a scholarship (tuition and books), the family does not receive any type of financial assistance regardless of how well the athlete is playing. NCAA rules state that prospective athletes beginning as early as the ninth grade cannot receive monetary benefits or gifts. This is applicable to family members and relatives of prospective intercollegiate athletes. Failure to comply with this rule will make the prospective athlete ineligible (Sanregret, n.d.). Although the NCAA boasts of providing more than 180,000 student athletes with over 3.5 billion dollars in annual scholarships, many of the athletes leave families struggling in poverty without community assistance. Thus, communities closely identify with athletes emerging from their communities because the community is considering future possibilities (giving back) from the athlete who grew up in their community. The community is morally supportive and welcomes the athlete with the expectation that the athlete will become a professional in the future.

Additional pressures are placed on athletes by fans (alumni and friends) who expect to see their college team win. When athletes do not win, fans stay at home, and this could mean loss of millions of dollars for the college. Therefore, the coaches are responsible for ensuring game wins. Coaches are replaced quickly if they do not produce a winning team. The game not only impacts the college or university, but also businesses that increase prices during game days and expand their restaurant menus, showcase team paraphernalia, and increase their tailgate inventories. The game is not simply "a game" to be enjoyed; it is big business that impacts the well-being of athletes, their families, fans, and the community.

SUMMARY

College athletics is big business in American society, bringing in billions of dollars to colleges and universities. However, are these institutions of higher learning failing these athletes and making them victims of a capitalistic enterprise? Potential athletes are scouted at a young age when their athletic abilities are displayed in middle school. By ninth grade they are recruited and offered a letter of intent by an institution of higher learning. They can either enter a college or university with a full scholarship (tuition, books, room and board) or if considered an elite status, the professional sport may offer a contract.

Some athletes such as Bryce Harper do not complete high school and enter the professional sports world at a very young age (16 on the cover of *Sports Illustrated*). He made his major league baseball debut at age 19. LeBron James was also recruited from high school and functioned in the NBA. Some spectators may suggest that he made the "right" choice, and this may be accurate. However, we can see the missing features of college life in flaws in his professional traits. For example, the camaraderie team spirit that college athletes share and take to professional sports teams is not visible in James as he boasts of his personal skills and degrades teammates and coaches he feels are not doing as he suggests.

College athletes are more prone to using alcohol, marijuana, and prescription drugs as their primary drugs of choice. Some of the consequences are increased injury rates, mental health issues (e.g., depression or suicide ideation), ineligibility (termination from the team which results in leaving college), and legal issues. Prevention and intervention strategies are limited to these athletes due primarily to stigma attached to "having problems" and discussing them with a counselor. The challenges for these college student athletes are known; research should determine how the numerous barriers can be overcome so that these athletes can receive desperately needed assistance. Until the college and university administrators, coaches, and players remember that the life of a player should outweigh the dollars, the ball and chain syndrome of college athletics will continue to exist.

DISCUSSION QUESTIONS

1. Explain what is meant by "college athletics is big business." This task can be accomplished by forming groups in the classroom to discuss the issue and either selecting one person to report back to the class the findings or the group submitting a short written explanation that can be used for extra credit. This focus can also be used for a class final paper assignment as well.
2. It is important to remember that all athletes are not the same, nor do they emerge from the same background. But they all have the urge to win. Discuss your thoughts about the NCAA's rules regarding ineligibility status. For example, what can cause athletic ineligibility?
3. The focus of this chapter is on issues related to drug use among college athletes. What factors may cause a college athlete to use illegal drugs?
4. Should coaches receive sanctions for athletes who become addicted to prescription drugs due to injury while engaged in their sport?
5. Current literature suggests that Greek fraternities are becoming as notorious as some street gangs (e.g., drug use and hazing). Should athletes be prohibited from becoming members of Greek life while on a sports team?

REFERENCES

Addiction Center. (2021). College students and drug abuse. Recovery Worldwide. https://www.addictioncenter.com/college/

Barry, A. E., King, J., Sears, C., Harville, C., Bondoc, I., & Joseph, K. (2016). Prioritizing alcohol prevention: Establishing alcohol as the gateway drug and linking age of first drink with illicit drug use. *Journal of School Health*, *86*(1), 31–38.

Chang, T. (2018). Are energy drinks with high caffeine okay for athletes? Shasta Orthopaedics Sports Medicine Team. https://shastaortho.com/shasta-orthopaedics-blog/are-energy-drinks-with-high-caffeine-okay-for-athletes/

Choo, T., Roh, S., & Robinson, M. (2008). Assessing the "gateway hypothesis" among middle and high school students in Tennessee. *Journal of Drug Issues*, *38*(2), 467–492.

Drug Enforcement Administration (DEA). (2021). Drug Scheduling & Classifications (List of Schedule–V Controlled Substances). American Addiction Centers. https://americanaddictioncenters.org/prescription-drugs/classifications

Golembeski, D. (2022). NCAA loosens marijuana rules for college athletes. Best Colleges. https://www.bestcolleges.com/news/2022/03/01/ncaa-loosens-marijuana-thc-policy/

Hainline, B., Bell, L., & Wilfert, M. (n.d.). Mind, body and sport: Substance use and abuse. NCAA. https://www.ncaa.org/sport-science-institute/mind-body-and-sport-substance-use-and-abuse

Hawryluk, M. (2019, December 27). America's marijuana growers are the best in the world, but federal laws are keeping them out of global markets. *The Washington Post*. https://www.washingtonpost.com/business/2019/12/27/americas-marijuana-growers-are-best-world-federal-laws-are-keeping-them-out-global-markets/

Karst, A. (2018, December). Weighing the benefits and risks of medical marijuana use: A brief review. *Pharmacy (Basel)*, *6*(4), 128. doi: 10.3390/pharmacy6040128.

Kirby, T., & Barry, A. E. (2012). Alcohol as a gateway drug: A study of US 12th graders. *Journal of School Health*, *82*(8), 371–379.

Lampe, J. (2021, February 5). The Controlled Substances Act (CSA): A legal overview for the 117th congress. Congressional Research Service. https://fas.org/sgp/crs/misc/R45948.pdf

Lopez, G. (2016, August 11). The federal drug scheduling system, explained. *VOX Media*. https://www.vox.com/2014/9/25/6842187/drug-schedule-list-marijuana

Memedovich, K. A., Dowsett, L. E., Spackman, E., Noseworthy, T., & Clement, F. (2018, July–September). The adverse health effects and harms related to marijuana use: An overview review. *CMAJ Open*, *6*(3), E339–E346. https://doi.org/10.9778/cmajo.20180023; https://www.ncbi.nlm.nih.gov/pmc/articles/PMC6182105/

Moore, M., & Abbe, A. (2021). The National Association of Intercollegiate Athletics Substance Use and Abuse Survey. *Journal of Issues in Intercollegiate Athletics*, *14*, 95–114.

NCAA. (2015). NCAA releases drug use study. https://training-conditioning.com/article/ncaa-releases-drug-use-study/

NCAA. (2017a). Drug testing program. https://www.ncaapublications.com/p-4608-2020-2021-drug-testing-program-booklet.aspx

NCAA. (2017b). What student-athletes need to know about marijuana. https://www.ncaa.org/sport-science-institute/topics/what-student-athletes-need-know-about-marijuana

NCAA. (2021). 2020–2023 NCAA banned substances. https://www.ncaa.org/sports/2015/6/10/ncaa-banned-substances.aspx

Salas-Wright, C. P., Vaughn, M. G., & González, J. M. R. (2016). Genetic underpinnings. In *Drug abuse and antisocial behavior* (pp. 53–72). Palgrave Macmillan.

Sanregret, J. (n.d.). *Houghton High School student athlete handbook*. https://www.hpts.us/Athletic_Handbook.pdf

Shakil, S. S. M., Gowan, M., Hughes, K., Azam, M. N. K., & Ahmed, M. N. (2021, March). A narrative review of the ethnomedicinal usage of Cannabis sativa Linnaeus as traditional phytomedicine by folk medicine practitioners of Bangladesh. *Journal of Cannabis Research, 3*(1), 8. doi: 10.1186/s42238-021-00063-3.

Skidmore, C., Kaufman, E., & Crowell, S. (2016, September). Substance use among college students. *Child and Adolescent Psychiatric Clinics of North America 25*(4), 735–753. https://www.researchgate.net/publication/307968152_Substance_Use_Among_College_Students

Substance Abuse and Mental Health Services Administration (SAMHSA). (2016, November). Facing addiction in America: The surgeon general's report on alcohol, drugs, and health [Internet]. Appendix D: Important facts about alcohol and drugs. U.S. Department of Health and Human Services. Office of the Surgeon General. https://www.ncbi.nlm.nih.gov/books/NBK424847/

Villa, L. (2019). How common is drug abuse among athletes and do they seek treatment? American Addictions Center. https://rehabs.com/addiction/among-athletes/

Weaver, E. D. V. (2020). *Agents of capital: The role of Black Greek letter fraternities in the experiences of Black men at predominantly White institutions* (Doctoral dissertation, Rutgers The State University of New Jersey, School of Graduate Studies). https://www.proquest.com/openview/10a8d1800bc7af2f4e6ce5b30defc19f/1?pq-origsite=gscholar&cbl=18750&diss=y

Professional Athletes and Issues Related to Drug Use

INTRODUCTION

In professional sports, athletes are often faced with a decision to use illicit drugs despite the risk that discovery of drug use can harm an athlete's career and have negative physical effects that follow the athlete after retirement. In the context of professional sports, illicit drug use can include the use of recreational drugs, opioids to mask pain, and performance-enhancing drugs, which is generally referred to as *doping*. Professional athletes use recreational drugs such as marijuana, cocaine, and heroin to reduce stress without inherently affecting performance (Dimeo, 2010, p. 33). Among professional athletes, opioid use often begins to deal with the pain associated with injury, but can become long-term use to maintain performance and dependence that may continue even after the end of a professional athlete's career (Cottler et al., 2011, p. 188). The performance-enhancing drugs involve steroids, which are synthetic versions of testosterone, and human growth hormones that enhance the development of muscle but can cause significant harm to the body from long-term use (Solberg & Ringer, 2011, p. 92). Estimates of the use of performance-enhancing drugs among athletes range from 10% to 40%, depending on the sport (Kabiri et al., 2020, p. 6).

The use of illicit drugs among professional athletes is influenced by complex economic, social, and personal factors that contribute to decisions made by the athletes. The following sections contain a discussion of the cultural factors, sense of victimization, family factors, community expectations, and fan pressure that can contribute to drug use among professional athletes. Questions for further discussion are presented at the end of the chapter.

CULTURAL FACTORS

Some evidence from research suggests that the sport culture can be a contributing factor for performance-enhancing drug use among professional athletes (Solberg & Ringer, 2011, p. 94). The culture of professional sports organizations is composed of a set of values and behavioral norms that create the context for athletes' decision making. The informal values and norms of professional sports organizations differ significantly from general social values concerning fair play and the norms of behaviors that should be used to defeat sport competitors. Professional sports organizations have an aggressive and competitive set of values, which influences athletes that are members of the organization. Consequently, professional sports teams adopt an informal culture that places the highest priority on winning and accepts or overlooks behaviors that involve aggression and even cheating, as long as the behavior contributes to the objective of winning. The informal culture encourages ego-driven behavior in which the self-interest of individual athletes and the desire to display dominance over others influences their decision-making process.

In many professional sports teams, the owners and managers of teams ignore the use of performance-enhancing drugs among athletes, which helps to legitimize the use of illicit substances as being tacitly accepted by the organization (Solberg & Ringer, 2011, p. 97). In some cases, officials such as managers or trainers procure performance-enhancing drugs for professional players, further embedding the use of drugs in the organizational culture. The attitude of the team toward performance-enhancing drugs implicitly communicates that these types of drugs are not so bad when compared to the damaging effects of alcohol, tobacco, or illegal recreational drugs (Kabiri et al., 2020, p. 10).

Sports culture can also encourage the misuse of opioids and other drugs to deal with pain from sports injuries. Injuries are common for professional athletes, with the severity of the injury often dependent on the type of sport (Cottler et al., 2011, p. 188). Professional teams place a substantial amount of pressure on athletes to recover from injuries as quickly as possible. In addition, the culture of professional athletes emphasizes the importance of dealing with pain to continue playing in competition (Murphy & Waddington, 2007, p. 242). As a result, professional athletes will often attempt to conceal the extent of an injury or the full scope of an ongoing problem with an injury through the use of opioids and other pain medications. Research by Cottler et al. (2011, p. 190) determined that 52% of professional football players in the United States use opioids during their careers, with 12% obtaining opioids exclusively from an illicit source. Approximately half of all players reporting the use of opioids also reported obtaining opioids from both physicians and illicit sources. The rationale for obtaining opioids from illicit sources was the need to continue playing the sport despite pain and to conceal the scope of the problem from the professional team. Pain that persists after retirement is also the rationale for professional athletes to continue misusing opioids and other pain medications.

A professional sport culture functionally creates an environment in which individuals seeking to participate in professional sports have to accept the norms and values of the culture. Aspiring professional players become aware of the norms concerning performance despite injury and the role of enhancing drugs, opioids, and other types of illicit drugs as they prepare to become professionals. Peer socialization is an important part of the process of learning about the norms and values associated with illicit drug use in professional sports and the demands placed on team members. Professional athletes that know a performance-enhancing drug user in sports are seven times more likely to use a performance-enhancing drug (Kabiri et al., 2020, p. 6). In effect, awareness of drug use among peers in professional sports and awareness of its toleration as part of sport culture has a significant influence on the decision of an athlete to use performance-enhancing drugs and opioids. At the same time, the culture normalizes the use of performance-enhancing drugs with anecdotal examples of professional athletes with long and successful careers who attribute their abilities to the use of performance-enhancing drugs and opioids in the event of an injury (Solberg & Ringer, 2011, p. 93).

Victimization

A strand of research that considers professional athletes as victims of the sports industry can contribute insight into the motivation for drug use among professional athletes. Professional sports have become highly commercialized with owners, sponsors, and media having an important financial stake in the performance of teams and individual athletes (Murphy & Waddington, 2007, p. 240). The commercial stakeholders have an implicit agreement with professional athletes that the athlete will be well compensated to deal with the physical risks inherent in the sport, as long as their performance meets professional standards. At the same time, many of the professional athletes understand that the high level of compensation is unavailable in any other type of work, and therefore consider it acceptable to offset the risk of physical injury. The relationship between financial stakeholders and athletes is fundamentally exploitive with the athlete as the victim, even in situations in which the compensation will end if the player is injured or does not perform in accordance with stakeholder expectations or standards. At the same time, athletes do not consider themselves victims. Nonetheless, the lack of control associated with victimization manifests itself among professional athletes as fear of losing a place on the team because of inadequate performance. The lack of control becomes a motivator for athletes to use performance-enhancing drugs to improve playing ability and opioids to mask pain as a means of placating the owner, sponsor, and media victimizers of the sports industry.

A high-pressure performance environment created by the sports industry can also contribute to the use of illicit drugs as a maladaptive means to reduce stress (Westberg et al., 2017, p. 95). Rather than deal with the sense of victimization that develops from the pressure to perform at high levels, some athletes turn to cocaine or other illicit substances as a means of relaxation and temporary escape. In some cases, professional athletes use both performance-enhancing drugs and other illicit substances at the same time, which compounds the physical risks associated with substance abuse. Research by Cottler et al. (2011, p. 93), for example, found that football players that used opioids as a means to continue playing despite significant injury also consumed large amounts of alcohol.

Family

The relationship of professional athletes with their family can influence their decision to use performance-enhancing drugs, as well as other drugs. A significant family factor contributing to the use of drugs among professional athletes is the expectations of family members for continued high performance of the athlete and career advancement. The desires and aspirations of family members are an important factor in the decision of many college athletes to turn professional (Carreathers, 2020). For some families, the possibility of a son or daughter earning a large salary from professional sports is a consideration for remaining in professional sports. Consequently, family pressures can easily contribute to the decision of professional athletes to use performance-enhancing drugs or to use opioids as a means of maintaining a position on a team. Family pressures can also create an indirect incentive for professional athletes to use drugs in order to be in a better position when negotiating salary with team owners.

Families can also influence the use of drugs among professional athletes through the behaviors and attitudes of other family members (Kabiri et al., 2020, p. 10). In social learning theory, family members influence the norms and behaviors of young people at least until adolescence. Some individuals that eventually become professional athletes learn early behaviors by imitation of the older members of the family. If illicit drug use of any kind is apparent in an older member of the family, a professional athlete is more likely to consider the behavior of using drugs as normal based on early childhood observations. Consequently, a professional athlete from a family with one or more users of illicit drugs is more likely to consider the use of performance-enhancing drugs, nonprescription opioids, or other types of drugs as acceptable behavior.

Community

Community expectations can place additional pressure on professional athletes to use drugs for enhancing performance and masking the pain associated with injuries. Many athletes come from minority communities and become role models for people in the community concerning the value of hard work, perseverance, and financial success in sports. As a result, the community expects professional athletes to maintain a high level of performance and to demonstrate good character (Westberg et al., 2020, p. 97). Community expectations for superior performance in sport and exemplary behavior in private life places substantial pressure on athletes to ensure they can live up to the expectations. Consequently, professional athletes that are sensitive to the expectations of their original community as well as the general sports community are more likely to use performance-enhancing drugs or opioids to maintain their standing as a valued professional athlete. In addition, the professional athletes are likely to make a substantial effort to conceal their use of illicit substances because of the possibility of diminishing their standing in a community.

Athletes that rely on illicit performance-enhancing drugs and nonprescription opioids to conceal pain often use other illicit substances in combination with recreational drugs (Dimeo, 2010, p. 32). In some cases, the pressure from the effort to conceal the use of drugs to improve performance leads to stress that the professional athlete addresses with the use of another substance, such as cocaine, which can lead to addiction. In addition, a professional athlete that uses recreational substances as an amateur player is more likely to consider using performance-enhancing drugs or opioids to lessen pain as acceptable behavior after becoming a professional.

Fans

Fans create an approach–avoidance situation for professional athletes with respect to performance-enhancing drugs and the use of opioids to overcome pain associated with injury. Fans place substantial pressure on players to function at the highest possible performance level at all times, which creates an incentive for the athlete to use drugs that can improve or maintain performance. Fans can create pressure through their comments about a professional player's performance in fan interviews, in blogs, and in social media. The formal media can also influence fans' attitudes towards a professional athlete with the tone and scope of coverage. Some professional athletes enjoy the attention provided by fans and will take steps to ensure that they perform in accordance with fan expectations.

Fan expectations for performance can contribute to legitimizing the use of performance-enhancing drugs among professional athletes (Solberg & Ringer, 2011, p. 95). In some sports, such as baseball, fans have long been aware of and accepted various practices, such as the use of corked bats to obtain an unfair advantage. As a result, some fans have an expectation that their favorite teams and athletes will use any means possible to win. The professional athletes interpret the support of fans as a need to use any means possible to win, including the use of performance-enhancing drugs. Some fans can be very forgiving towards professional athletes revealed to have used performance-enhancing or other types of drugs (MacPherson & Kerr, 2019, p. 9).

Despite the implicit acceptance of drug use among professional athletes and among some fans, other fans adopt a more critical position when the drug use by the professional athlete becomes public knowledge. The change in fan attitudes toward athletes discovered to have used performance-enhancing drugs may be the result of negative media coverage and frequent public criticism of the athlete's behavior (MacPherson & Kerr, 2019, p. 3). The changeable nature of fans and the public shaming of athletes that have used drugs create a strong incentive for professional athletes to conceal illicit drug use from the public.

SUMMARY

The information in the previous sections supports the conclusion that many factors influence the decision of professional athletes to use illicit drugs to improve or maintain performance or enjoy the recreational aspects of the drug. Various factors contribute to the rationalization process of the athlete when making the decision to use a drug. Athletes often convince themselves that the only way to continue in professional sports is through the use of drugs.

The culture of professional sports is highly competitive and aggressive and emphasizes the importance of continuing to play despite the pain resulting from injury. The competitive and aggressive culture fosters the use of performance-enhancing drugs, while the attitude toward pain encourages the use of opioids. Sports culture also implicitly tolerates the use of performance-enhancing drugs and opioids, while publicly condemning the practice.

The perspective of the professional athlete as the victim of the club owners, sponsors, and media as stakeholders in the sports industry can also influence drug use among professional athletes. Although the athlete generally receives a substantial salary, the stakeholders have the expectation that the player will perform according to professional standards at all times. To meet these expectations, professional athletes often use performance-enhancing drugs to build muscle and stamina and opioids to continue playing despite pain.

The player's family can also pressure a professional athlete to be successful, which can influence use of performance-enhancing drugs and opioids to continue playing. The social learning that occurs in a family can also predispose an athlete toward the use of drugs. Community expectations for athletes create pressures for performance that can lead to the use of drugs. Fans have expectations for their favorite athlete's performance that contribute to legitimizing the use of drugs from the perspective of the athletes. Fans, however, can abandon a professional athlete once the athlete's use of illicit drugs becomes public knowledge. Athletes need support to withstand all these pressures.

DISCUSSION QUESTIONS

1. How can professional sports teams address the problem of drug use among professional athletes?
2. What is the relationship between amateur and collegiate athletes using drugs and drug use among athletes who play professionally?
3. How should professional athletes who are discovered using performance-enhancing drugs or opioids not prescribed by a doctor be sanctioned by the sports team or the league?
4. How do professional athletes that do not use drugs treat athletes that do use drugs?
5. Should any action be taken against teams that implicitly tolerate the use of performance-enhancing drugs or nonprescription use of opioids?

REFERENCES

Carreathers, B. (2020). Athletes' substance abuse and mental health. *MacNair Scholars Research Journal, 13*(1), 1–14. https://commons.emich.edu/mcnair/vol13/iss1/3/

Cottler, L., Abdallah, A., Cummings, S., Barr, J., Banks, R., & Forchheimer, R. (2011). Injury, pain, and prescription opioid use among former National Football League (NFL) players. *Drug and Alcohol Dependence, 116*(1–3), 188–194. https://doi.org/10.1016/j.drugalcdep.2010.12.003

Dimeo, P. (2010). Understanding and managing drugs in sport. *The Shield-Research Journal of Physical Education and Sport Science, 5*, 29–43. https://sujo-old.usindh.edu.pk/index.php/THE-SHIELD/article/view/996

Kabiri, S., Shadmanfaat, S., Howell, C., Donner, C., & Cochran, J. (2020). Performance-enhancing drug use among professional athletes: A longitudinal test of social learning theory. *Crime and Delinquency,* online publication in advance of print, 1–25. https://doi.org/10.1177/0011128719901111

MacPherson, E., & Kerr, G. (2019). Sport fans' responses on social media to professional athletes' norm violations. *International Journal of Sport and Exercise Physiology,* published online ahead of print, 1–18. https://doi.org/10.1080/1612197X.2019.1623283

Murphy, P., & Waddington, I. (2007). Are elite athletes exploited? *Sport in Society, 10*(2), 239–255. https://doi.org/10.1080/17430430601147096

Solberg, J., & Ringer, R. (2011). Performance-enhancing drug use in baseball: The impact of culture. *Ethics and Behavior, 21*(2), 91–102. https://doi.org/10.1080/10508422.2011.551466

Westberg, K., Stavros, C., Smith, A. C. T., Newton, J., Lindsay, S., Kelly, S., Beus, S., & Adair, D. (2017). Exploring the wicked problem of athlete and consumer vulnerability in sport. *Journal of Social Marketing, 7*(1), 94–112. https://doi.org/10.1108/JSOCM-07-2016-0035

Theoretical Perspectives Explaining Athletes' Behavior

INTRODUCTION

Everyone has a theory about something. However, when it comes to human behavior, theory is extremely important, and practitioners must use theory to guide their practice. Therefore, to simply state that an athlete continues to miss games because of arrogance is an insufficient explanation. To indicate that an athlete should not drop out of high school and sign with the pros because the athlete needs an education is not a sufficient explanation. There is a need to explore, explain, and be able to predict behavior based on theoretical soundness, as opposed to emotional explanations. Emotional explanations are based on personal attributes (values, attitudes, and experiences), whereas theory is based on evidence-based practice (what has been proven by researchers and practitioners to be effective when working with clients). Theory provides an empirical approach to explaining behavior. Theory has been utilized in psychology, social work, mental health, and addiction counseling as a framework for explaining human behavior. Numerous textbooks are written on theory; however, few provide suggestions on application. In other words, how do you link theory to what the client is experiencing in their world (environment) that may be extremely complex and unimaginable? Working with athletes presents a different convergence of explanations in their complex environment. Therefore, there is a need to consider all dimensions of not only their human behavior, but also their social environment.

The inclusion of all theoretical perspectives in this chapter is an unreasonable task. The aim is to include theories from social work, psychology, criminal justice, and sociology that are considered dominant theories to explain human behavior. When these theories are understood, any other theoretical domain can be used to explain social, psychological, and biological aspects of human behavior while recognizing them from the point of strengths and limitations. You may be thinking, *but how can we explain the NCAA from this social, psychological, and biological perspective?* Macro-level theories are also discussed with examples provided. Often students become bored or even frustrated with theory classes because they cannot understand the relevance when they are told to memorize theories and theorists. The suggestion here is not to memorize but to understand how to actually apply the theories.

WHY IS THERE A NEED TO STUDY THEORY?

Theory guides social work practice. It allows the clinician to describe, explain, and predict behavior (Thomas, 2017). The use of theory is a major best practice aspect of clinical practice (person-in-environment). However, the focus is expanded in this chapter to encompass not only the individual, but also communities, groups, organizations, and families because these entities are significant when explaining theory that focuses on athletes. There is a need to study theory because there is a need to understand the hows and whys of behaviors, and theoretical conceptualizations provide that component.

Theories also allow clinicians to protect their license by depersonalizing and become more objective with their assessments. Depersonalizing allows the practitioner to move away from their value system and focus on the client's value system. In this manner, biased clinical practice is terminated, or at least reduced. Information guided by theory is less likely to cause harm to the client and to the practitioner because the practitioner is relying on theory to support the thinking in the client's file.

Another reason to study theory is that it provides language that other practitioners will understand. For example, when assessing a case and the practitioner indicates that the client is experiencing some unresolved childhood experiences brought on by childhood traumatic incidents, most practitioners will quickly relate this to Freudian psychodynamic theory. So understanding theory allows for a universal language in practice. Theories guide the social work process by assisting with the formation of questions, development of treatment plans, and design of intervention strategies. Theories provide the foundation or framework for analyzing the client's problem. Practitioners engaged in research are also theory bound in that their research, qualitative or quantitative or applied, as they rely on theory to explain their observations that cannot be sufficiently interpreted without a theoretical basis. Therefore, it is extremely important for practitioners to know, understand, and apply theories when working with clients, organizations, communities, and families.

For our purposes in this chapter, *theory* is defined loosely as basic assumptions. However, in social sciences, theory is an empirical entity that is designed to answer the question of why and can provide explanations and predictions about human interactions and behaviors. There has been concern among researchers regarding a generation gap in theoretical thinkers (generation theorists fading) (Wallace, 2017). The suggestion is that every 25 years there should be a new set of theoretical perspectives. The Chicago School, for example, provided leadership in the production of theoretical outlooks focused on socialization, as opposed to the notion that heredity dictates individual behavior. After the Chicago School, the emergence of studies based on personality traits became significant due to the continuing wars and PTSD as a major focus of treatment for those who served in the military. It has been noted that there are few theoretical perspectives that focus on the technology age of cell phones and computers. However, limited theoretical discussions have focused on technology and social change, which Ogburn termed "cultural lag theory."

This chapter on theories provides a cursory delineation of basic theoretical perspectives. "Basic" here implies mainstream (theories that are well known and recognized in the field of social sciences). In addition, models, methods, and approaches are also identified because often they are used interchangeably and discussed as theories even when there are basic differences. Using the ATM perspective to outline the differences, we begin with A as the approach to the situation. Before meeting with the client, after review of the client's file, thinking about how and where to begin is a key factor in establishing rapport.

Next, T represents theory applied as the social worker begins to understand the client's situation and identify the problem. Finally, M means model and will include discussions regarding methods and skills to intervene. The preference may be individual counseling sessions initially. The ATM perspective allows the creation of an understanding between the theory approaches, methods, and models so that it is clear to the social work intern the differences between the cognitive and skills levels of practice. In-depth information is not discussed because this is not a theory textbook. But sufficient information is offered so that the ATM perspective can be understood and applied to athletes as the reader deems appropriate.

Theory can be divided into major categories: sociological, psychological, biological, and critical theories. Many theorists group theories together based on categorized features (biological, psychological, or sociological); therefore, in this chapter, basic theoretical examples will be provided utilizing the broad categories.

SOCIOLOGICAL THEORIES

Sociological theories support the notion that behavior is impacted by individual and environmental factors and allow us to explain the why of the interaction of things. Sociological theories focus on the links or connections between human behavior and environmental factors. For example, the Chicago School suggested the need to focus on communities and their organization. Their findings suggest that social disorganization has an impact on human behavior. Typically, sociological theories are categorized into three main categories: structural functionalism, conflict theory, and symbolic interactionism. For our purposes, broad categories of micro (individuals) and macro (society) levels will be the focus because the theories are constantly evolving (Davis, 2016) and subcategories become less stressful when students master the broad categorical theoretical perspectives.

Symbolic Interaction Theory (aka Symbolic Interactionism)

Although Herbert Blumer is the sociologist who coined the phrase symbolic interactionism in 1937 (Cole, 2019), it was George Herbert Mead is who is attributed with in-depth critical thinking between "I" and "me" that lead symbolic interaction theory to its highest pinnacle (Crossman, 2020). Other sociologists used Mead's work to enhance and create other aspects of the theory. Charles Horton Cooley, for example, expanded on Mead's work and can be seen in the 21st-century selfie movement ("I" sending selfies to make "me" so that I can be seen by everyone) (Cole, 2019). In other words, Cooley was saying that self-perceptions influence actions. So, athletes act a certain way (wearing their athletic clothes) because that is the way they perceive themselves (and they want to influence others by wearing the athletic clothes and by also walking on campus with other team members).

According to symbolic interaction theory, reality is a social construct based on the social interactions within social contexts (Cole, 2019). Interpretation of communication is accomplished through symbols. Athletes wear athletic gear on campus to symbolize their affiliation with sports. When they are not wearing their sports gear, they wear other clothing to symbolize their status, such as designer caps, clothing, and tennis shoes. These symbols express to the campus that they are special and their lifestyle is different than other students on campus. These symbols reaffirm their elite status and signify to those they encounter that they are members of a powerful group on campus. They act and react based on not only the athletic interpretation of their world, but also based on how they are viewed or interpreted. Therefore, when the athlete walks on campus, they are revered and treated graciously by all, especially if they are winning games, and even more so if they are the team star.

Mead's thinking was further expanding by Cooley with his looking-glass explanation, which is a cognitive component of interaction theory. He suggested that imagination plays a large role in how we view ourselves as we consider how others view us. For example, an athlete may think that because they are a star athlete, they possess certain rights and privileges. This is true in the athletic department; however, there may be a different perspective of the athlete outside of the athletic department. Regardless of the environment, the athlete's behavior can be explained using theory to support the explanation.

Social Learning Theorists

Social learning theorists believe that behavior is learned based on interactions. For example, **Albert Bandura** (1925–2021) used Bobo dolls to prove his thinking regarding the observation and imitation analogy. He suggested that behavior is learned by observing the behavior of others and then imitating that behavior. View the Bandura experiments with the dolls at YouTube.

Edwin Sutherland (1883–1950) was a firm believer in social learning and suggested that peers learn criminal behavior from other peers through interactions based on similar values, goals, and attitudes. He called his theory Differential Association. He formulated nine principles (propositions) of social learning. View the videos on Sutherland's contribution to social learning theory at YouTube.

Travis Hirschi (1935–2017) formulated the social bonding theory (aka social control theory) identifying four areas that impact behavior positively or negatively. Those four areas—(1) attached, (2) commitment, (3) involved, and (4) belief—will impact how a person behaves. He suggested that when the bond is broken, even in one of the areas, there will be behavioral changes. The focus is on how strong ties to the four areas can reduce the likelihood of negative consequences.

Robert Merton (1910–2003) argued that the American dream places strain on individuals to accomplish because not everyone has the resources to accomplish, and therefore, the strain causes negative consequences (e.g., criminal activity, health issues, even suicide). Merton further stated that when opportunities or resources are blocked, a state of anomie emerges and individuals become creative to design methods of accomplishing their goals.

PSYCHOLOGICAL THEORIES

Psychological theories, unlike sociological theories, focus on internal factors such as emotions, feelings, motivations, personalities, and cognitive processing, using conscious and unconscious thoughts to explain behavior. Psychological theories are categorized into six grand theories: (1) psychoanalysis, (2) behaviorism, (3) cognitivism, (4) humanism, (5) ecological, and (6) evolutionary. However, all of these theories will not be covered extensively in this chapter.

Psychoanalysis

Psychoanalysis credits Freudian thinking. **Sigmund Freud** (1856–1939) is considered the father of psychodynamic theory as he believed that the unconscious mind was a major factor in understanding human behavior and explaining why individuals behaved in a certain manner. He formulated features of the human personality into the id, ego, and superego. He suggests that the id is an impulsive or instinctive reactive action that seeks immediate gratification. It has aspects that are both destructive, non-pleasant, (aggressive behavior/violence) and positive (eating, breathing). While the ego is used as part of a conscious and unconscious process, its goal is to satisfy the needs of the id in a manner that is acceptable by societal norms. It is termed the *reality principle*. The superego informs the ego of the need to function in a morally acceptable way. It functions as if policing behaviors, instructing what is right and wrong. These elements of Freudian personality theory are based on the premise that they may not act in tandem (together). For example, an athlete may desire to use drugs at a fraternity party (id), but, the players may be reminded that they will be kicked off the team (superego) if they use so they can then decide to leave the party and not engage in drug use (strong ego). However, if the decision is to remain at the party and use drugs, the superego loss the battle of encouraging the right thing to do (leave the party and do not use drugs to remain on the team).

Freud is considered the grandfather of psychosexual theory, which is used by many family and marriage counselors in practice. He firmly believed that sexual drives (id) were key features to explaining and describing human behavior. Freud believed that personality was formed at age five and behavior displayed following this age is a result of the personality developed. His development of the psychosexual model is grounded is sexual orientations, with each stage of development representing a sexual body part (Kassel, 2020). The five stages are oral, anal, phallic, latent, and genital.

Although there is conflict suggested in each of the stages, Freud suggested that resolving the conflict can move the individual smoothly to the next stage. However, some individuals may not resolve the conflict, leaving the unresolved conflict to continue and affect the individual later in life. He suggested that unresolved conflicts may occur as a result of fixation (being stuck) in the stage, which could result in an unhealthy personality (Cherry, 2022).

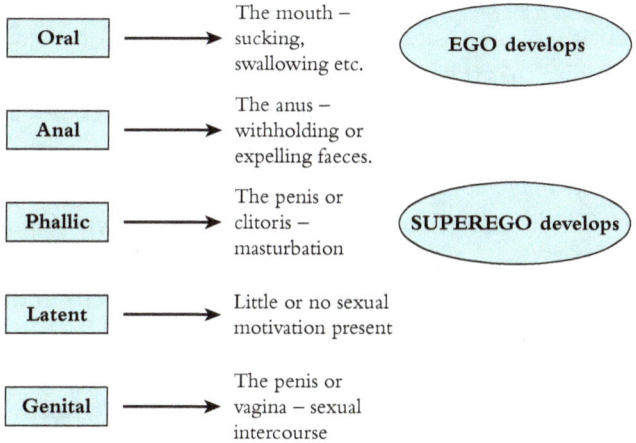

FIGURE 4.1 *Psychosexual Stages of Development*

Erik Erikson (1902–1994) stood on the shoulders of Freud and formulated a life span development model with the suggestion that it is important to view human behavior from beginning (infancy) to end (elderly). Like Freud, Erikson believed in personality theory and the development of psychosocial stages of development. However, Erikson developed three additional stages than Freud's five stages of psychosexual development, suggesting that positive and negative behavioral experiences exist on a continuum and impact personality.

TABLE 4.1 **Erikson's Eight Stages**

Stage	Psychosocial Crisis	Basic Virtue	Age
1.	Trust vs. Mistrust	Hope	0–1½
2.	Autonomy vs. Shame	Will	1½–3
3.	Initiative vs. Guilt	Purpose	3–5
4.	Industry vs. Inferiority	Competency	5–12
5.	Identity vs. Role Confusion	Fidelity	12–18
6.	Intimacy vs. Isolation	Love	18–40
7.	Generativity vs. Stagnation	Care	40–65
8.	Ego Integrity vs. Despair	Wisdom	65+

Source: McLeod, S. (2019). Erik Erikson's stages of psychosocial development. Simply Psychology. https://www.simplypsychology.org/Erik-Erikson.html

At each of the eight stages, there is a crisis that should be resolved. As the crisis situations are resolved, the development of an empowered individual emerges. However, if the crisis is not resolved, more problematic issues can occur. Other life span development theorists such as Piaget and Kohlberg focused on the mental processing of development.

Cognitivism Theory

Jean Piaget's (1896–1980) theory on intelligence (cognitive development) suggested that children learn differently than adults and that their learning style can be assessed in the four stages of cognitive development that he posed: sensorimotor, preoperational, concrete operational, and formal operational.

Piaget felt that individuals learn based on their experiences as it relates to their understanding. Experiential learning was considered a key factor in understanding because the cognitive process changes over time as individuals mature. These changes occur as a result of social experiences, biological maturation, activity, and equilibration. For example, it is important for children to play with each other because the play helps them to develop and advance their cognitive processes to understand abstract concepts. **Lev Vygotsky** (1896–1934) agreed with Piaget to an extent. He suggested that it was not all experiential learning that increased knowledge but that a knowledgeable person teaching is the missing link that Piaget did not include in his thinking regarding cognitive development. Vygotsky suggested that culture and language are crucial factors in the cognitive process. Therefore, social interactions enhance cognition in humans. He deviated from Piaget's thinking that the stages were applicable to everyone

TABLE 4.2 Piaget's Four Stages

Stage	Age	Characteristics	Goal
Sensorimotor	Birth to 18–24 months old	Motor activity without use of symbols. All things learned are based on experiences, or trial and error.	Object permanence
Preoperational	2 to 7 years old	Development of language, memory, and imagination. Intelligence is both egocentric and intuitive.	Symbolic thought
Concrete operational	7 to 11 years old	More logical and methodical manipulation of symbols. Less egocentric and more aware of the outside world and events.	Operational thought
Formal operational	Adolescence to adulthood	Use of symbols to relate to abstract concepts. Able to make hypotheses and grasp abstract concepts and relationships.	Abstract concepts

Source: Marcin, A. (2018).

as he emphasized the notion that cultures are different and individuals in different cultures experience the cognitive stages of development differently. His focus was on language, culture, and the role of the community in cognitive development.

Moral Stages of Development

Lawrence Kohlberg (1927–1987) followed in the footsteps of Piaget with the thinking that there are "fixed" stages that individuals experience in moral reasoning. Moral reasoning or morality focuses on what is right and what is wrong based on societal norms. In his cognitive–ethical model of reasoning (Snarey, 2012), Kohlberg explained how moral behavior is developed by delineating three levels with two stages at each level of moral reasoning. The levels are preconventional, conventional, and post conventional. Each of these stages has two sublevels that provide an understanding of ethics and morality as he focused on justice.

Level 1: Preconventional (sense of morality and obedience)

> Stage 1: Punishment orientation where there is a desire to obey the rules to avoid punishment. Children (ages 4–10) respond to external controls (e.g., parents, teachers, authority figures) because they understand morality to mean doing what adults explain that you should do.
>
> Stage 2: Instrumental orientation focused on "what's in it for me" or "scratch my back" with the thinking that individual best interest is a key factor in this stage.

Level 2: Conventional (sense of morality)

> Stage 1: Good boy and nice girl orientation—seeking the approval of others.
>
> Stage 2: Law and order orientation is the key feature, with an intent to obey the rules even if they are not viewed as reasonable.

Level 3: Post Conventional (morality becomes an abstraction—laws should be changed)

    Stage 1: Social contract orientation considering differences and allowing different opinions.

    Stage 2: Universal orientation with the emphasis on ethical principles and the primary focus on equality, dignity, and respect. The thinking, according to Kohlberg, is that the laws are valid if there is a justice framework.

Like all theories, Kohlberg's moral development theory was closely scrutinized. Many disadvantages have been listed for not using his theory, such as Gilligan's writing that Kohlberg's theory on moral development is androcentric and his focus on justice does not include the "ethics of care" performed by females. The suggestion that moral reasoning for males is more advanced than for females has not been scientifically proven. But we do know that both males and females respond to reward and punishment in similar patterns.

Operant Conditioning

Burrhus Frederic (B. F.) Skinner (1904–1990), on the other hand, thought that learning occurs primarily as a result of responses to stimuli. This thinking is based on the reward and punishment continuum. Positive behavior is rewarded while negative behavior is punished. This type of learning, termed operant conditioning, is based primarily on associations. Skinner described operant conditioning as behaviors that occur as a result of the events (stimuli) that impact the behaviors (reinforcement). For example, when athletes perform well in their sport (stimuli), they receive cheers from the crowd, acclaims from the coach, and large professional contracts to play in professional sports (reward). The positive reinforcement of a professional contract stimulates the athlete to continue to perform well. However, punishment is also a consideration in the operant conditioning paradigm. If college athlete misses a practice game due to oversleeping, the coach may remove the athlete from the roster for the next two games as punishment. This negative reinforcement (removal from the next two games) is used to stimulate the athlete to refrain from missing practice games. Skinner suggested that both positive and negative reinforcements can be used to change behaviors. The change can occur as a result of cognitive processing or physical or biological attributes such as genetics.

BIOLOGICAL THEORIES

Biological theories suggest that human behavior occurs due to predetermined means and that the individual has limited or no control because of the hereditary trait. It is based on the reasoning that parents or genetics influence behavior and, therefore, little can be done to eliminate the genetic tracks. The main focus of biological theories is to consider how genetic factors impact behavior. **Charles Darwin** (1809–1882) is often the individual who is attributed to linking genetics to behavior, suggesting that behaviors occur beyond the individual's control. According to Darwin, all life is related, and due to natural selection, species will change over time, only to be replaced by newer forms (Hayden, 2009). Spencer is said to have coined the phrase "survival of the fittest" (Falk, 2020), which is rooted in the thinking of social Darwinism (the idea that rich individuals deserve to be rich and poor individuals deserve to be poor based on natural selection). Darwin's thinking is still relevant in contemporary society.

Theories of Heredity

Johann Gregor Mendel (1822–1884) is considered the father of genetics as he was the first to explain that children inherit their appearances from their parents. As he expanded on Darwin's theory, Mendel suggested that evolution starts with genes. Using pea plants to test his theory, he concluded that genes come in pairs and genetic composition is a key factor in the natural selection process as different traits in humans cause competition and struggles among each to survive. Mendel's theory was applied to humans and useful in seeking cures for diseases. However, Mendel's theory has been used to justify trying to create a superior race, as was the objective in Hitler's Germany. In America, eugenics uses political, economic, and social venues to impose racial prejudices on individuals and groups, suggesting that only the strong (White Americans) should survive and the weak (minorities) will get what is coming to them. However, in America the issue becomes muddled because the majority of the weak (welfare recipients) are the White dominate population.

Cesare Lombroso (1835–1909), like Mendel, believed that individuals inherit their characteristics from their parents. However, Lombroso connected the physical characteristics to crime as he suggested that certain types of individuals commit crimes. He described the appearance of those individuals as having large ears, sloping or receding forehead, and an asymmetric face (Wickert, 2020). Lombroso published a book in 1876, *The Criminal Man*, that described in detail the physical characteristics of the born criminal. He suggested that these born criminals are evolutionary backward individuals, functioning in a primitive state (atavists) where they emerged from a line of ancestors who carried the criminal gene. That gene can appear within a generation in the family. He noted that these family members can be identified by primitive physical and mental traits. Unlike Mendel and others who based their theories on experiments with plants and or insects, Lombroso studied human characteristics (offenders, nonoffenders, and mentally ill), measuring their bodies and recording the information while working in an Italian prison setting as a prison doctor. Schneider (2014) as cited by Wickert (2020) lists the primary focus of Lombroso's theory:

- The criminal can be distinguished from the noncriminal by numerous physical and psychological anomalies.
- The criminal is a variety of the human species, an anthropological type, a degenerative phenomenon.
- The criminal is an atavism, a "degeneration" to a primitive, subhuman type of human being. Criminals are modern "savages," physical and mental setbacks to an earlier stage of human history, to phylogenetic past. Criminals display physical and psychological characteristics that were believed to have been overcome in the history of development.
- Crime is inherited; it arises from a criminal disposition. (Schneider, 2014, p. 322)

Theory of Body Type

Lombroso inspired others to consider the role of body type when explaining human behavior. **William Sheldon** (1898–1977), standing on the shoulders of Lombroso, stated that body types are inherited, and he delineated three specific body types to explain criminal behavior: endomorphs, ectomorphs, and mesomorphs. Suggesting that the body type is linked to personality to prove his theory, he developed a classification system (somatotyping) that provided detailed descriptors for each body type. Endomorphs have lots of body fat, weight problems and gain weight easily. This category of body types are characterized as enjoying food, sociable, fun, even tempered, relaxed, and affectionate. Most football lineman fall into this category. Ectomorphs have long thin bodies with a flat and delicate appearance, introverted personality, and limited or poor social skills. They are self-conscious, private, artistic, and thoughtful. Many basketball players fall into this category. Mesomorphs are muscular and sturdy with broad shoulders. They are neither too fat nor too skinny and can seemingly control their weight as they are considered to be well proportioned. They are competitive, risk takers, assertive, do not care what others think, bold, and seek dominance. Most athletes fall into this category. Maddan et al. (2008), stimulated by Sheldon's work, suggested a need to focus research on body mass index (BMI) as a more useful and credible method of obtaining information linking anatomical type connections to behavior.

Similar to racial profiling, body type profiling should be cautioned against. Sheldon's somatotyping theory stimulated other researchers to either prove or disprove his theory. For example, Arthur Jensen and Charles Murray argue that heredity (genetic differences) does play a major role in explaining and predicting behavior. However, they focused on mental capacity, suggesting a gap between the races with some races (White) having a higher mental capacity (IQ) than other races (Black) (Woo, 2012).

CRITICAL THEORETICAL PERSPECTIVES

Critical theories are grounded in a macro perspective with the thinking that societal changes can bring about individual changes. They challenge the status quo and seek to stimulate critical thinking about issues related to social, political, and economical societal structures. A primary goal is to seek social justice for all citizens. Although **Max Horkheimer** (1895–1973) is credited with the development of critical race theory, most researchers and students quickly associate the name Karl Marx with critical theory.

Karl Marx (1818–1883) focused on capitalists and the working class, suggesting that there is a constant struggle and conflict between the haves (rich and powerful) and the have-nots (working class and poor and powerless) in society. His theory was that without social justice, the working class would eventually obtain power and take control. Considered the father of communism, he focused primarily on economic control that would provide a classless society, in comparison to capitalism that enhances inequality in society and causes ongoing conflict and struggles between the different classes. He believed that a classless society would achieve the greatest good for everyone. Marx's ideas have been said to describe the negative nature of capitalism (Thompson, 2019). Yet Marxist approach may be gaining some ground in the United States because lethal killings by police officers of unarmed Black males continues to be an issue in need of immediate reform.

Feminist Theory

Feminist theory is categorized in the conflict theorist's paradigm with a focus on gender issues related to power, dominance, and oppression. Gender differences can be viewed from a biblical framework, beginning with Adam and Eve in the garden of Eden. From a religious perspective, the agreement is that Eve was created from one of Adam's ribs, signaling the first level of inequality as Eve had to be thankful to Adam for her existence whereas Adam only had to praise and thank God for his existence. Throughout the 17th and 18th centuries, women maintained a subservient demeanor to their male counterparts. Although numerous women throughout history advocated and demonstrated that they could perform equal to men, it was not until the 1848 Seneca Falls convention that Elizabeth Cady Stanton took the lead to declare rights for women, which started the American women's rights movement (Frost-Knappman & Cullen-DuPont, 2004). Although White middle-class women lead the movement, they sought consultation from emanate male slaves such as Frederick Douglass and abolitionist Henry B. Blackwell, who strongly encouraged the women in the movement to seek political inclusion (Marilley, 1996). Although these White women were elite (upper-class wealth), they strongly advocated for change based on egalitarian dimensions in society, which is termed liberal feminism. For example, female players and coaches earn much less money than their male counterparts.

Radical feminist theory has a similar focus as liberal feminist theory on gender differences; however, the message is slightly different. Catharine MacKinnon and Andrea Dworkin are the most vocal radical contemporary feminists who argue that societal norms are the perpetrator of female oppression, intimidation, and abuse by males as a result of socially constructed ideas and roles based on gender. Dworkin suggests that pornography and date rape are illustrations of male dominance over women, treating women as mere sex objects. They advocate for criminalizing male intimidation and oppression of women. MacKinnon suggests that power is male power and gender socialization is based on the female identification of sex roles or existing for men's sexual pleasures (MacKinnon, 2019). MacKinnon (2019) provides a graphic portrayal of White women in her explanations for feminists advocating to change laws and punish men who oppress women. The change of laws to criminalize male behaviors that dominate and suppress women supports her theory that male domination is the causal factor for explanations of the way women behave in a patriarchal society. She further distinguishes between the way White women are treated and the manner in which minority women are treated by males, both Blacks and Whites, indicating that White women—although considered by both White and Black males as delicate and fragile in need of protection—are still treated as sexual objects. This she equates with slavery.

White Privilege

White privilege is seldom discussed in classes on theory because many of the students in the classes are White and many of the professors are White. Therefore, they do not want to feel uncomfortable or guilt-ridden. However, McIntosh (1989) suggests that there is a need to discuss White privilege to sensitize Caucasians to the extent of their power and the impact that it has on individuals, groups, laws, policies, and infrastructures. McIntosh lists more than 35 things she does not have to consider simply because she is White. Her theory is that different rules apply to those who are White in America. She termed these rules an "invisible knapsack" for Whites only. For example, she states that she does not have to train her children how to react when they see a police officer. When she goes for a job interview she can be assured that the interviewers will be White. She states that she can go shopping in a store and not have to fear being followed or harassed for suspicion of stealing. She notes that she can turn on the television or movie or open a newspaper at any time and see her White race represented in very positive manners. She can compete in sports and do well without it being said that she is a credit to her race. McIntosh's (1989) list continues as she indicates that many Whites take daily conditions for granted, never have to consider their safety as an issue. In addition, Whites do not have to consider these issues as problematic for other individuals or groups—they do not have to consider the issues at all because what is seen in society is "normal" and a pattern that has been passed on through generations by Whites due to unearned power (McIntosh, 1989).

Unearned power is bestowed by birthright or as a consequence of reward resulting from an encounter such as war or revolution. White skin in America is conferred dominance and unearned entitlement. Her remedy is to not only continue to view individual acts of racism as illegal, but also to begin securitizing invisible racism within systems and dismantling the democratic myth that there is equality for all Americans in America. It is difficult to give up power and dominance, and as McIntosh suggests, systemic change is a long, gradual process (McIntosh, 1997, p. 298). However, acknowledgement that there is White privilege can be a beginning (McIntosh, 1997, p. 299). Then follows the willingness to apply equality to all American citizens, regardless of race, religion, or national origin, as stated in the constitution. Privileges are not conferred to some individuals and groups or by one dominate group in power.

Critical Race Theory (CRT)

Derrick Bell (1930–2011) is credited with formulating critical race theory. CRT had its beginnings in 1989 in Madison, Wisconsin, when a group of scholars (Derrick Bell, Richard Delgado, and Alan Freeman) met at a convent to discuss concerns that the civil rights movement of the 1960s had stalled (Delgado & Stenfancic, 2017) and there was need to continue to address the issues, especially legal issues, related to ongoing racism in American society. As a result of that meeting the CRT was created, and today it has expanded to include diverse disciplines and diverse groups (e.g., Asian, Latino, Muslims, feminists, and Native American scholars). CRT suggests that race or racism is the core of issues related to social justice in America. Although it provides explanations for behavior—how America aligns itself along racial lines—it also provides strategies for change (Delgado & Stenfancic, 2017). The basic tenets of CRT as delineated by Delgado and Stenfancic (2017) include the following:

- First, racism is the basis of American society and a daily experience by the majority of people of color, although not acknowledged by the dominate group (Whites) unless blatant discrimination is displayed (such as mortgage redlining).
- The second tenet is material determinism, which allows for some legal successes if they benefit Whites, such as the Brown decision to integrate public schools. Bell suggested that *Brown v. Board of Education* [1956] was useful not out of a sense of right or wrong but a sense of self-interest for elite White liberals.
- The third theme of CRT delineated by Delgado and Stenfancic (2017) is social constructionism suggesting that race is constructed by societal norms that were not inclusive of people of color. The concept of race is based on created categories and has little scientific value based on intelligence, personality, or motivation.
- The fourth tenant is differential racialization, which means that popular images and stereotypes of groups shift over time, depending on their utility.

CRT purports that racism is normal and embedded in American society and changes or modifies only when there is need by the dominate society. This thinking, as with other theories, has sparked criticism of the thinking as socialism, pessimism, and anti-American (Bell, 2018; Delgado & Stefancic, 1993; Karimi, 2021). Tennessee and Idaho banned the teaching of critical race theory (CRT) from public school curricula as a Marxist ideology and a threat to the American way of life (Karimi, 2021). CRT, similar to White privilege, is seldom discussed in theory classes of higher education. However, there has been a need to revisit the theory amidst the current climate in America following the George Floyd murder by police officer Derek Chauvin on May 25, 2020. Although former officer Chauvin was found guilty of manslaughter, the atmosphere in the country continues to focus on race as a critical variable in oppressive behaviors. Critical race theorists suggest that race is engrained in the fabric of American society and impacts relationships, thought, and quality of life. Race is common, institutional, and gives Whites an advantage in the legal system (Bell, 2018). CRT is considered an academic movement that views American society and legal issues from a race perspective and has received not only controversial criticism and attacks (Cobb, 2021) but has been banned from teaching in some states (e.g., Tennessee, Florida, Idaho, Arkansas, Oklahoma, and New Hampshire). There are currently other states with legislation to also ban the teaching of CRT in public schools. The map can be viewed at https://worldpopulationreview.com/state-rankings/states-that-have-banned-critical-race-theory.

MODELS: THERAPEUTIC INTERVENTIONS

The words *models* and *theories* are sometimes used synonymously; however, theories provide plausible explanations for behavior while models describe how theories can work. A few of the popular models will be described, but, this is not an exhaustive list of models. Some of the models that will be described are Afrocentric, biosocial, strengths, CBT, narrative, motivational interviewing, brief therapy, death/dying, aversion, conversion, dialectical, and crisis intervention. Wunsch (1994) suggested that theories and models have a blurred connection that can overlap, but models provide the "how to" (application) component of theories. Models enhance the understanding of theories by providing instructions on how to apply theories. Most theories help describe, explain, and predict behavior, but they do not suggest what to do or how to do it.

Models help us intervene. Both theory and model are essential in social sciences. How do they connect and relate? What approach will be used? Maclean (2020) provides a clear distinction between theory, model, and approach in the social sciences and encourages students to not only understand that these concepts are connected, but how they differ in practice. Consider theory as a means to provide understanding of behavior, model as schematic structure that puts forth the intervention strategy to clarify the understanding (theory), and approach as the personal style (technique) that is used to implement the intervention strategy (model). For example, social workers are familiar with Freudian psychodynamic theory. The strategy (model) is to uncover unresolved childhood traumatic experience. The approach can differ based on the individual social worker's techniques used in practice. All social workers will understand the theory and the model, but the techniques used (approaches) will depend on different variables (e.g., client, setting, policies, social worker's value and belief system). A simple model for conceptualizing these concepts follows:

Theory = understanding; model = intervention strategy; approach = technique(s)

Theory = understand

Model = structure – intervention strategy

Approach = technique

Let's examine a few examples of models and approaches.

Strength-Based Perspective

Dennis Saleebey (1936–2014) is often credited with the strength-based approach in practice. Saleebey (2006) suggested that clients will be better helped if therapists focus on the client's strengths (e.g., resources, interests, goals, and personal characteristics), as opposed to focusing on pathological factors such as the client's weakness or institutional failures. The client can resolve their problems with assistance from a therapist when the client has a stronger sense of self-confidence and self-awareness, and a feeling of empowerment. The therapist's primary role is to assist the client in understanding their resilience and their ability to bring about change. This strength-based approach is grounded in ecological and social construction theory (Anderson & Heyne, 2013).

The Disease Model of Addiction

Elvin Morton (E. M.) Jellinek (1890–1963) is considered the father of the addiction model. The disease model of addiction is the perspective that an addiction is an illness that can be treated, but not cured. The thinking is that the individual who is addicted does not choose to be addicted, but the addiction causes large brain surges of dopamine in the brain, which, in turn, causes more and more need for the dopamine surges in order to function and creates an endless cycle of continual addiction (NIDA, 2015). This model is grounded in biological and genetic theoretical perspectives. Lesser (2021) suggests that 87%

TABLE 4.3 Jellinek's Four Stages of Addiction Model

Pre-Alcoholic Stage	The problem often comes from people drinking for social reasons and who start drinking to relieve stress or to feel better.
The Prodromal Stage	Middle stage of drinking during which the drinker begins to have blackouts and continues to drink alone and in secret while their alcohol tolerance increases.
The Crucial Stage	Type of alcoholism that is characterized by frequent drinking. It can also cause visible alterations to the victim's brain and body.
Chronic Stage With Daily Drinking	Alcohol as the main focus of life, physical and mental issues with long-term alcohol abuse, and health problems cropping up from alcohol misuse.

Source: Lesser, B. (2021, April 14). Alcoholism: The disease theory. Dual Diagnosis.org. https://dualdiagnosis.org/alcohol-addiction/disease-theory-alcoholism/

TABLE 4.4 Prochaska and DiClemente's Six Stages of Change Model

Stage 1. Precontemplation	In this stage, people do not intend to take action in the foreseeable future (defined as within the next 6 months). People are often unaware that their behavior is problematic or produces negative consequences. People in this stage often underestimate the pros of changing behavior and place too much emphasis on the cons of changing behavior.
Stage 2. Contemplation	In this stage, people intend to start the healthy behavior in the foreseeable future (defined as within the next 6 months). People recognize that their behavior may be problematic, and a more thoughtful and practical consideration of the pros and cons of changing the behavior takes place, with equal emphasis placed on both. Even with this recognition, people may still feel ambivalent toward changing their behavior.
Stage 3. Preparation (Determination)	In this stage, people are ready to take action within the next 30 days. People start to take small steps toward the behavior change, and they believe changing their behavior can lead to a healthier life.
Stage 4. Action	In this stage, people have recently changed their behavior (defined as within the last 6 months) and intend to keep moving forward with that behavior change. People may exhibit this by modifying their problem behavior or acquiring new healthy behaviors.
Stage 5. Maintenance	In this stage, people have sustained their behavior change for a while (defined as more than 6 months) and intend to maintain the behavior change going forward. People in this stage work to prevent relapse to earlier stages.
Stage 6. Termination	In this stage, people have no desire to return to their unhealthy behaviors and are sure they will not relapse. Since this is rarely reached, and people tend to stay in the maintenance stage, this stage is often not considered in health promotion programs.

Source: LaMorte, W. W. (2019, September 9). The transtheoretical model (stages of change). Boston University School of Public Health. https://sphweb.bumc.bu.edu/otlt/mph-modules/sb/behavioralchangetheories/BehavioralChangeTheories6.html

of American adults have consumed alcohol at some point in their lives. NCAA cautions athletes about drinking after a winning game to celebrate because alcoholism is usually progressive and is considered a fatal disease. Therefore, controlled and regulated drinking is prescribed if abstinence is not achieved (Clark, 2016). If drinking and taking other drugs become an addiction, intervention strategies can include the Jellinek four disease stages and the six stages of change drug model developed in the late 1970s by Prochaska and DiClemente.

Each of these addiction models provide intervention techniques that can be applied when working with clients during the different stages.

Cognitive Behavioral Therapy (CBT)

Cognitive behavioral therapy (CBT) grounded in cognitive theory is a popular therapeutic intervention that is used in different practice settings. CBT is said to have been developed by **Aaron T. Beck** (1921–2021) who is known as the father of cognitive therapy. Beck suggested that negative behavior should be changed to positive behavior, and this change could occur as a result of changing the cognitive (thought) processes. Therefore, the focus should be on the client's thoughts, beliefs, attitudes, and perspectives. To change the thinking patterns of the client, the worker should focus on the thinking that is creating the problem and assist the client with restructuring and reframing their thoughts. This restructuring can be accomplished using different techniques, such as journaling, storytelling, miracle questions, and listing things that make the client happy. These techniques can be accomplished during the session or as homework assignments that can be discussed in a session and continued as an ongoing process. The goal is replacement of negative thoughts with positive thoughts, or thoughts that are more productive (realistic and useful) for the client's well-being. CBT can be used in settings with children, adolescents, and adults (Sukhodolsky et al., 2004) with mental disorders and physical problems (Wenzel et al., 2016) or illicit drug use and alcohol addiction (Magill & Ray, 2009).

Motivational Interviewing

Motivational interviewing (MI), developed by William Miller and Stephen Rollnick, is grounded in person-centered theory and has been found useful when working with clients experiencing substance use disorders, chronic pain or disease, obesity, or diet and exercise adjustments. Miller and Rollnick (2002) delineated the principles and the basic approach of MI. These principles include (a) **empathy**—viewing the client's world as the client sees it; (b) **self-efficacy**—believing that the client can change; (c) **roll with resistance**—believing that the counselor should not impose their thoughts onto the client and "solve" the problem for the client; and (d) **develop discrepancy**—assisting the client to understand how the client's problematic behavior/attitude may hinder them from accomplishing their goal(s).

A basic approach used in MI is called OARS. The acronym stands for **Open-ended questions** and allows clients opportunity to express their thoughts and provide the counselor with more insight into the client's perspective change continuum; **Affirmations**, which evoke honest positive traits or behaviors voiced by the client, demonstrating to the client strengths that they may not have perceived; **Reflections**, a demonstration to clients that what they are saying is being understood by reviewing some of the core elements of the client's conversation; and **Summaries**, which includes the counselor providing a gist of the session delineating key factors for the shift to change. The OARS represent the methods that should be used by counselors practicing MI. Specific examples of questions by the counselor can be found using the SAMSHA Treatment Improvement Protocol (TIP) (SAMSHA, 1999).

Brief Therapy

Unlike MI, brief therapy (aka solution focused) is a solution-focused therapeutic intervention that is counselor directed. The focus is on the present problem and specific behaviors. Brief therapy or solution-focused brief therapy was developed by **Steve de Shazer** (1940–2005) and **Insoo Kim Berg** (1934–2007). It is strength-based with attention to clients' goals and the focus on the solution and how to maintain the solution so that the problem does not reoccur (Corcoran & Pillai, 2009). Brief therapy is grounded in cognitive behavioral and psychodynamic theories (Groves & Blais, 2008).

Brief therapies should include the following characteristics, according to SAMSHA, tip number 34 (1999):

- screening and assessment,
- core assessment areas,
- initial session,
- treatment goals,
- subsequent sessions,
- maintenance strategies,
- ending treatment, and
- follow-up.

This short-termed intervention relies on techniques such as miracle questions, scaling questions, and doing things differently. Although clients can change and have the resources for bringing about change, they are guided by the therapist.

Moral Model

The moral model has foundations in Kohlberg's cognitive thinking regarding moral development. Moral model focuses on what is good and bad and punishment and reward (D'Andrade, 1995). It is the opposite of the disease model, where the thinking is that the individual's genetics or heredity is the major element in the disease. The individual is the primary focus in the moral model as the person who knows right from wrong and is responsible for their actions. The goodness and badness of the behavior is subjective and measured by the individual's character. The moral model focuses on individual choice and considers the individual who succumbs to substance use disorder as weak, with the ability to discontinue. Grounded in social learning theory, the perception is that the individual learned to use alcohol and other substances.

Harm Reduction Model

Harm reduction model is a set of strategies and ideas developed to reduce the harm of risky behaviors. It is also considered a social justice movement with the establishment of the National Harm Reduction Coalition. It is designed to reduce the risky illicit or illegal behaviors by imposing strategies that lessen the punitive consequences for the behaviors. Harm reduction model started as a movement in the 1970s by activists (doctors, grassroots people, social scientists, and policy makers) to reduce the punitive consequences of individuals who use drugs (Roe, 2005).

In the 1980s the HIV/AIDS epidemic emerged and risky behaviors (with both sex and drugs) were at the forefront of public health issues. No longer were marginalized populations (drug using populations) the only victims, but HIV/AIDS was impacting all socioeconomic classes, both heterosexual and homosexual individuals. As a result, harm reduction became an attentive strategy for public health advocates. The focus is on helping clients engaged in risky behaviors to experience less harm and to have access to services. The harm reduction model, although considered a controversial model, has been proven to be an effective method of practice grounded in cognitive behavioral theories (Wright et al., 2012).

This model is considered a liberal approach to drug use, allowing or permitting the use of drugs but designed to reduce and, if possible, eliminate the punitive consequences of drug use (Marlatt, 1996).

Basic principles of the harm reduction model (NHRC, 2021) overlap with basic assumptions. The assumptions are that a public health alternative to the moral or criminal and disease model of drug use and addiction is a better option for individuals and society as a whole. Although abstinence is the overall goal, an effective option is knowing alternatives to reduce harm that are beneficial to the quality of life of many individuals engaging in risky behaviors.

According to the National Drug Alliance (2021), the major harm reduction issues include the following:

- Drug overdose, which is considered the leading cause of drug deaths in the U.S. for drug users under the age of 50.
- Naloxone is a generic drug used to reverse the opioid overdose. It is FDA approved and inexpensive. However, fewer citizens have access and more training of professionals are needed to promote the use of Naloxone.
- Good Samaritan laws, which provide drug users with immunity from criminal sanctions if they call 911 for help. The notion is to get life-saving help for someone who may be overdosed on illicit drugs. Often other drug users or citizens who do not want to get involved will fail to call 911 due to fear of negative consequences from law enforcement or the court system.
- Syringe access to lower the risk of HIV and Hepatitis C. Limits syringe sharing and provides safe disposal options. Advocates for ending policies that criminalize syringe possession.
- Drug checking supports policies to distribute drug testing supplies and equipment, allowing clients to identify the drug(s) used to reduce the dangerous unknown drugs contaminating products, such as fentanyl. The education of drug users regarding "bad drugs" (those laced with other chemicals) is an effective strategy to minimize the deaths.
- Advocating the need for supervised consumption services, as in the Netherlands where facilities are available for users to use drugs in supervised areas in order to reduce overdose deaths. These overdose prevention facilities are designed to permit on-site supervised drug use. Currently, the closest analogy to this in the U.S. is provided by the states that have decriminalized marijuana use, and Oregon is the only U.S. state that has decriminalized all drugs for personal use.

Advocates of the harm reduction model, such as the National Harm Reduction Coalition, continue to express and develop ideas and strategies that can be used by counselors to work with policy shifts such as the decriminalization of risky behaviors.

Death/Dying Model

Elisabeth Kübler-Ross (1926–2004) developed a five-stage model of death and dying. This model is significant because every human being will die, and yet it is seldom discussed in theory classes. Addicted clients are especially vulnerable to death and dying due to their personal issues and need for assistance in resolving those issues. Corr (2020) poses interesting questions regarding the usefulness of Kübler-Ross's work in contemporary society in higher education. The argument here is the reality that everyone will die or grieve at some point in time, and this model provides a framework for counselors to not only assist clients, but also to recognize and become willing to openly and honestly discuss issues related to death, dying, and grieving. The five stages of dying and grief according to Kübler-Ross (1969) include the following:

Denial—experiencing thoughts of "this cannot be true" or feeling of numbness, which is the body's natural defense mechanism to assist with survival while dealing with loss.

Anger—this is a natural response that will dissipate. Anger can include lashing out at family members, friends, and even deities (higher powers) for the loss.

Bargaining—this is the negotiation stage or the "what if stage" of the loss process and includes trying to make deals to improve the situation in instances of illness ("Make the person better, and I will do …") or blaming self ("If only I had taken them to see a doctor sooner").

Depression—feelings of emptiness and not wanting to do anything but think about the loss. Isolation and not wanting to interact with others. In some instances, suicide ideation may emerge with feelings of not wanting to continue living with the loss.

Acceptance—the realization that a traumatic change has occurred, but there is need to continue on to remember the times enjoyed. Good memories will replace the emptiness of the loss.

Kübler-Ross suggested that these stages are sequential and can be overcome (Editors of Psycom, 2021). However, if a client is experiencing difficulty coping with the loss, counseling will be an effective option to assist the client to move successfully to the acceptance stage.

SUMMARY

Theories about human action(s) can be classified under one of the three broad categories—biological, sociological, or psychological—or there may be an overlapping of theoretical perspectives (biopsychosocial) to explain and predict behavior. Theory is used to guide not only theoretical research, but also to guide social work practice. Therefore, to downplay, limit the use, or not discuss theory is a major error in discussions about human behavior. Ignatow (2020) argues that there is a lack of theoretical innovation now, as we tend to be moving in a downward slope. Turner, Hicks, and Zucker (2019) identify a generation gap in theorizing, speculating that this gap could be due to the digital age. If this gap is considered a theoretical crisis gap, is technology the cause? Or are we experiencing a state of stagnation due to enormous changes in academia? Or is there a new generation of millennial intellectuals who are seeking to change the connections of society (Harker et al., 2016). Whether theory is in a state of crisis or a temporary state of stagnation, theory is an essential component of understanding human behavior at the micro and macro levels of practice.

Is theory relevant in today's technological world? Theory is necessary for understanding and predicting human behavior. It is needed to make sense of the world (Halford & Savage, 2017). A major advantage for utilizing theory is that it is evidence-based (scientifically proven) as a useful tool providing universal understanding when explaining behavior. Theory provides probabilistic predictions that can lead to effective problem-solving when working with athletes. If environmental factors can be identified early, and intervention strategies (models of practice) implemented timely, the probability of the athlete experiencing negative outcomes will be greatly reduced.

DISCUSSION QUESTIONS

1. Discuss why theory is important to know and understand.
2. Why do college/university athletes behave the way they do? Use theory to support responses.
3. Discuss the differences between a theory and an approach, model, and method. Provide examples. Review the YouTube video titled "What is the difference between a theory, model, method, and approach in social work?"

    https://www.youtube.com/watch?v=nE1rKczA2kk
4. Every theory has its strengths and limitations. Select a theory and explain the strengths and then identify some limitation.
5. Explain why you think a specific college athlete behaved a certain way. Then use a theory to support your thinking about the athlete's behavior.

REFERENCES

Adams, J. (2021). *Redeeming Justice: From defendant to defendant, my fight for equity on both sides of a broken system.* Convergent Books.

Anderson, L. S., & Heyne, L. A. (2013). A strengths approach to assessment in therapeutic recreation: Tools for positive change. *Therapeutic Recreation Journal, XIVI*(2), 89–108. https://bctra.org/wp-content/uploads/tr_journals/3873-13443-1-SM.pdf

Bell, D. (2018). *Faces at the bottom of the well* (Rev. ed.). Basic Books.

Cherry, K. (2022, July 27). Freud's psychosexual stages of development. Developmental Psychology. *Very Well Mind.* https://www.verywellmind.com/freuds-stages-of-psychosexual-development-2795962#:~:text=During%20the%20five%20psychosexual%20stages,as%20a%20source%20of%20pleasure.

Clark, N. (2016, December 6). The athlete's kitchen: Alcohol & athletes. *Sport Science Institute.* NCAA. https://www.ncaa.org/sport-science-institute/topics/athlete-s-kitchen-alcohol-athletes

Cobb, J. (2021, September 13). The man behind critical race theory. *The New Yorker.* https://www.newyorker.com/magazine/2021/09/20/the-man-behind-critical-race-theory

Cole, N. L. (2019). Symbolic interaction theory: History, development, and examples. *Thought Co.* https://www.thoughtco.com/symbolic-interaction-theory-p2-3026645

Corcoran, J., & Pillai, V. K. (2009). A review of the research on solution-focused therapy. *British Journal of Social Work, 39*(2), 234–242. doi:10.1093/bjsw/bcm098; https://www.researchgate.net/publication/240591088_A_Review_of_the_Research_on_Solution-Focused_Therapy

Corr, C. A. (2020, December). Elisabeth Kübler-Ross and the "five stages" model in a sampling of recent American textbooks. *Journal of Death and Dying, 82*(2), 294–322. https://doi.org/10.1177/0030222818809766; https://journals.sagepub.com/doi/10.1177/0030222818809766

Crossman, A. (2020). Biography of sociologist George Herbert Mead. *Thought Co.* https//www.thoughtco.com/George-herbert-mead-3026491

D'Andrade, R. (1995). Moral models in anthropology. *Current Anthropology, 36*(3), 399–408. https://www.unl.edu/rhames/courses/current/dandrade.pdf

Delgado, R., & Stefancic, J. (1993, March). Critical race theory: An annotated bibliography. *Virginia Law Review, 79*(2), 461–516. doi:10.2307/1073418. https://www.jstor.org/stable/1073418?seq=1

Delgado, R., & Stefancic, J. (2017). *Critical race theory.* New York University Press.

Editors of Psycom. (2021). The five stages of grief: An examination of the Kübler-Ross model. Psycom. https://www.psycom.net/depression.central.grief.html

Falk, D. (2020). The complicated legacy of Herbert Spencer, the man who coined "survival of the fittest." *Smithsonian Magazine.* https://www.smithsonianmag.com/science-nature/herbert-spencer-survival-of-the-fittest-180974756/

Frost-Knappman, E., & Cullen-DuPont, K. (2004). *Women's suffrage in America: An eyewitness history.* Facts on File.

Groves, J. E., & Blais, M. A. (2008). Brief psychotherapy: An overview. In T. A. Stern, J. F. Rosenbaum, S. L. Rauch, M. Fava, & J. Biederman (Eds.), *Massachusetts General Hospital comprehensive clinical psychiatry* (pp. 141–150). https://www.sciencedirect.com/sdfe/pdf/download/eid/3-s2.0-B9780323047432500135/first-page-pdf

Halford, S., & Savage, M. (2017). Speaking sociologically with big data: Symphonic social science and the future for big data research. *Sociology, 51*(6), 1132–1148. https://doi.org/10.1177/0038038517698639

Harker, R., Mahar, C., & Wilkes, C. (2016). *An introduction to the work of Pierre Bourdieu: The practice of theory.* Springer.

Hayden, T. (2009, February). What Darwin didn't know. *Smithsonian Magazine.* https://www.smithsonianmag.com/science-nature/what-darwin-didnt-know-45637001/

Ignatow, G. (2020). *Sociological theory in the digital age.* Routledge Publisher. https://doi.org/10.4324/9780429292804

Kassel, G. (2020). What are Freud's psychosexual stages of development? *Healthline.* https://www.healthline.com/health/psychosexual-stages

LaMorte, W. W. (2019, September 9). The transtheoretical model (stages of change). Boston University School of Public Health. https://sphweb.bumc.bu.edu/otlt/mph-modules/sb/behavioralchangetheories/BehavioralChangeTheories6.html

Lesser, B. (2021, April 14). Alcoholism: The disease theory. Dual Diagnosis.org. https://dualdiagnosis.org/alcohol-addiction/disease-theory-alcoholism/

MacKinnon, C. (1989). *Toward a feminist theory of the state.* Harvard University Press.

MacKinnon, C. (2019). *Butterfly politics.* Belknap Press.

Maclean, S. (2020, March 19). What is the difference between a theory, model, method and approach in social work? https://www.youtube.com/watch?v=nE1rKczA2kk

Maddan, S., Walker, J. T., & Miller, J. M. (2008). Does size really matter? A reexamination of Sheldon's somatotypes and criminal behavior. *The Social Science Journal, 45*(2), 330–344. https://www.researchgate.net/publication/256158341_Does_size_really_matter_A_reexamination_of_Sheldon's_somatotypes_and_criminal_behavior

Magill, M., & Ray, L. A. (2009). Cognitive behavioral treatment with adult alcohol and illicit drug users: A meta-analysis of randomized controlled trials. *J. Stu Alcohol Drugs, 70*(4), 516–527. https://pubmed.ncbi.nlm.nih.gov/19515291/

Marcin, A. (2018, March 29). What are Piaget's stages of development and how are they used? *Healthline.* https://www.healthline.com/health/piaget-stages-of-development

Marilley, S. (1996). *Women suffrage and the origins of liberal feminism in the United States, 1820–1920*. Harvard University Press.

Marlatt, G. A. (1996). Harm reduction: Come as you are. *Addictive Behaviors, 21*(6), 779–788. https://www.sciencedirect.com/science/article/abs/pii/0306460396000421

McIntosh, P. (1997). White privilege and male privilege: a personal account coming to see correspondences through work in women's studies. In R. Delgado & J. Stefancic (Eds.), *Critical White studies: Looking behind the mirror* (pp. 291–299). Temple University Press.

McIntosh, P. (1989, July/August). White privilege: Unpacking the invisible knapsack. *Peace and Freedom*, 10–12. https://psychology.umbc.edu/files/2016/10/White-Privilege_McIntosh-1989.pdf

McLeod, S. A. (2019, July 18). Erik Erikson's Stages of Psychosexual development. *Simply Psychology*. https://www.simplypsychology.org/psychosexual.html

Miller, R., & Rollnick, S. (2002). *Motivational interviewing: Preparing people for change* (2nd ed.). Guilford Press.

National Drug Alliance. (2021). *Building the bridge. Annual report*. https://drugpolicy.org/sites/default/files/dpa-2021-annual-report.pdf

National Harm Reduction Coalition (NHRC). (2021). Principles of harm reduction. https://harmreduction.org/about-us/principles-of-harm-reduction/

National Institute on Drug Abuse (NIDA). (2015, June 12). Addiction is a disease of free will. https://archives.drugabuse.gov/about-nida/noras-blog/2015/06/addiction-disease-free-will

Roe, G. (2005, September). Harm reduction as paradigm: Is better than bad good enough? The origins of harm reduction. *Critical Public Health, 15*(3), 243–250. http://www.harmreductionactioncenter.org/HRAC_DOCUMENTS/HARM%20REDUCTION%20--GENERAL/Origins_of_Harm_Reduction.pdf

Saleebey, D. (Ed.). (2006). *The strengths perspective in social work practice* (4th ed.). Allyn & Bacon.

SAMSHA. (1999). Motivational interviewing as a counseling style. In Center for Substance Abuse Treatment. *Enhancing Motivation for Change in Substance Abuse Treatment*. Substance Abuse and Mental Health Services Administration (U.S.). Report No. (SMA) 99-3354. https://www.ncbi.nlm.nih.gov/books/NBK64964/; https://www.ncbi.nlm.nih.gov/books/NBK64964/

Snarey, J. (2012, January). *Lawrence Kohlberg: Moral biography, moral psychology, and moral pedagogy*. Psychology Press. https://www.researchgate.net/publication/259982080_Lawrence_Kohlberg_Moral_biography_moral_psychology_and_moral_pedagogy

Sukhodolsky, D. G., Kassinove, H., & Gorman, B. S. (2004). Cognitive-behavioral therapy for anger in children and adolescents: A meta-analysis. *Aggression and Violent Behavior, 9*(3), 247–269. https://www.sciencedirect.com/science/article/abs/pii/S1359178903000727

Thomas, J. E. (2017). Scholarly views on theory: Its nature, practical application, and relation to world view in business research. *International Journal of Business and Management, 12*(9). https://pdfs.semanticscholar.org/6ae1/4dece731e4d72bbcba0de0b4e141cfedbfd1.pdf

Thompson, M. J. (2019). The radical republican structure of Marx's critique of capitalist society. *Critique: Journal of Socialist Theory, 47*(3), 391–409. doi.org/10.1080/03017605.2019.1642987; https://www.tandfonline.com/doi/abs/10.1080/03017605.2019.1642987

Turner, K., Hicks, T., & Zucker, L. (2019). Understanding how adolescents encounter, evaluate, and engage with texts in the digital age. *Reading Research Quarterly, 55*(7). doi:10.1002/rrg.271. https://www.researchgate.net/publication/334944657_Connected_Reading_A_Framework_for_Understanding_How_Adolescents_Encounter_Evaluate_and_Engage_With_Texts_in_the_Digital_Age

Wallace, W. (Ed.). (2017). *Sociological theory*. Routledge.

Wenzel, A., Dobson, K. S., & Hays, P. A. (2016). *Cognitive behavioral therapy techniques and strategies*. American Psychological Association. https://doi.org/10.1037/14936-000

Wickert, C. (2020, November 30). Lombroso's criminal anthropology. *Soz Theo*. https://soztheo.de/theories-of-crime/biological-theories-of-crime/lombrosos-anthropological-anthropogenetic-crime-theory/?lang=en

Woo, E. (2012, November 2). Arthur Jensen dies at 89; his views on race and IQ created a furor. *Los Angeles Times*. https://www.latimes.com/local/obituaries/la-me-arthur-jensen-20121102-story.html

Wright, T. E., Schuetter, R., Fombonne, E., Stephenson, J., & Haning, W. F. (2012, January 19). Implementation and evaluation of a harm-reduction model for clinical care of substance using pregnant women. *Harm Reduction Journal. 9*(5). https://doi.org/10.1186/1477-7517-9-5; https://harmreductionjournal.biomedcentral.com/articles/10.1186/1477-7517-9-5

Wunsch, G. (1994). Theories, models, and data. *Demografie, 36*(1), 20–29. PMID: 12346076. https://pubmed.ncbi.nlm.nih.gov/12346076/

IMAGE CREDIT

Fig. 4.1: Source: https://www.simplypsychology.org/psychosexual.html.

Intersection of Race, Gender, and Nationality in Sports

INTRODUCTION

Athleticism has been a valued trait in human beings since the dawn of the species. Some anthropologists believe, for example, that our ability to run for long distances was one thing that marked the transformation from hominid into modern man. The ancient Greeks held contests of athleticism and sport called the Olympic Games, which are held every four years to this day. To many then and many now, sport is not just about entertainment or passing time; it is about participating in or bearing witness to a testament to human physical prowess. It is about pushing the limits of the human form, the human mind, and the human spirit.

HISTORICAL LOOK AT COMPETITIVE SPORTS

The history of competitive sport is a long and storied one. However, like many elements of society and culture, sports have changed with the times. Games once attended casually in person are now broadcast across the world on television and radio waves, and often on their own tailor-made and sport-specific cable stations. In some Olympic sports, competition between amateur or semi-pro athletes has been replaced by competition between professionals who eat, sleep, and breathe the sport they play and are paid handsomely for it. Professional sports themselves have intensified in the last many decades. Athletes are paid more than ever before, and, indeed, compete to an unprecedented level. Athletes are spending more time training, dieting, and practicing in an effort to achieve their athletic goals.

While opinions on any sport-related topic are almost universally split, many feel that the exponential increase in competition in recent years has made watching sports more entertaining. Many idolize athletes on a personal as well as professional level, wearing jerseys with their player's names and following their exploits religiously. Many sports figures during the last century and beyond have achieved the status of legends in culture. In fact, the term *Ruthian*, used commonly to describe prodigious accomplishment in a particular field, comes from the name Babe Ruth, perhaps one of the most revered sports figures in American sports culture.

AFRICAN AMERICANS IN SPORTS

Sports have surely changed since Ruth's days. Ruth was overweight and an avid drinker and smoker—big taboos in today's world of fierce competition, where every athlete is doing everything possible to gain even the slightest potential physical edge over an opponent. In fact, baseball in recent years has been marred by steroid abuse scandals. Crucially, too, Babe Ruth played before African Americans were allowed to participate in the major leagues.

That is one of the universally positive changes to occur in sports in recent times—increased inclusivity. In 1947, Jackie Robinson famously became the first Black player to participate in the major leagues. More soon followed, and now most rosters in professional baseball are made up of mostly non-White players. This confirmed what many had long suspected—that the African American comprised Negro leagues held as much talent, if not more, than the major leagues. Other sports integrated in the years to follow, and many professional sports are now dominated by non-White players (Borish & Gems, 2000).

WOMEN IN SPORTS

Though women have long participated (though usually in separate categories) in certain sports—and all-female teams replaced men's minor league baseball teams during World War II (Borish & Gems, 2000)—a major step forward for women's equality in sports came in 1972, when Congress passed the education amendments. The amendments prohibited sex-based discrimination in any school that receives federal money. This had a massive impact on collegiate-level sports programs, and the National Collegiate Athletics Association, or NCAA, soon began including female athletics championships alongside male championships (NCAA.org).

Inclusion in college-level sports had a secondary impact on professional sports, as more and more women grew up playing sports and achieving athletically at a higher level. In 1997, the Women's National Basketball Association played its first game (WNBA.com). The last few decades have seen the formation of more professional or semi-professional women's sports leagues, including the United States Women's Football League in 2010 (Facebook.com/USWFL) and the National Women's Hockey League in 2015 (NWHL.zone). Women have not only demanded increased participation in professional sports, but increased compensation as well. In 2007, long-standing tennis Wimbledon Championships began offering equal prize purses for the men's and women's tournaments respectively, noting that viewership for and interest in women's championship matches often equaled or exceeded viewership for and interest in men's matches (Bodo, 2018).

RACISM AND SEXISM IN SPORTS

While participation in organized sport is as open to all comers as it has ever been, racism and sexism are still rampant in our society. This is reflected by much of the social and political upheaval of recent years. And though non-White and non-male athletes are now able to seize opportunities they may once have been denied, these athletes still face many struggles professionally and socially that their White male counterparts do not. This becomes especially relevant as sports and sports figures play an increasingly major role in society, culture, and even politics. The NFL, for example, has come under fire recently for using racist team mascots, as well as the treatment of one-time star quarterback Colin Kaepernick, who has remained unsigned for several seasons after protesting racial discrimination by kneeling during the nation anthem.

Women, too, face unique challenges in sports these days. Tennis star Serena Williams recently participated in, dominated, and was victorious in the Australian Open tournament while eight weeks pregnant. This stirred controversy and sexist backlash, with some admiring her play and others admonishing her for not taking time off.

The stressors of sexism and racism, explicit and implicit, affect not only athletes at the highest levels, but many non-White and non-male athletes participating at every level. A 2017 study conducted by the University of Lisbon in Portugal determined that among a sample group of 405 Portuguese athletes, female competitors had a greater fear of failure, and a greater embarrassment and "devaluat[ion] one's self-estimate" associated with such a failure (Correia et al., 2017). This reflects a commonly noted societal trend of over-confidence in achievement for men and an under-confidence of achievement for women.

While societal assumptions of failure can be harmful to athletes and female athletes in particular, societal assumptions about success can be harmful too. Author John Milton Hoberman writes in his book, *Darwin's Athletes: How Sport Has Damaged Black America and Preserved the Myth of Race*, "black identity is athleticized through ubiquitous role models who stimulate wildly unrealistic ambitions in black children (an improbable number of black boys expect to become professional athletes)" (Hoberman, 1997, p. 4). The main thrust of Hoberman's book attacks the commonly held notion that African Americans are superior athletes, noting that this assumption pushes many Black youth toward sport and away from achievement in other arenas, putting an emphasis on physical, performative value over intellectual or personal value, which harkens back to the assumptions about race made during the times of slavery (Hoberman, 1997).

Adding to Hoberman's point is the fact that while sporting organizations often tend to be made up of predominantly Black athletes, the front-office, coaching, and other organizational positions of power are still often held by Whites. A 2014 study of racial discrimination of athletes on college campuses notes that "Although there is an overrepresentation of African American athletes, the decision-making duties found in such occupations as ownership, leadership, and management positions are still largely occupied by White males" (Beamon, 2014). The study goes on to conclude that the African American male student athletes surveyed faced discrimination in numerous ways, not just in the form of institutional stereotyping and lack of opportunity but also at the hands of supposed fans, who, the study notes, "seemed to feel a sense of entitlement and did not hesitate to use racial descriptions, as well as racial epithets, to insult athletes when they fell short in competition" (Beamon, 2014).

The issues of pain and injury attitudes are also becoming increasingly relevant to all athletes in recent times, as more and more research indicates that playing through certain types of injury can lead to traumatic long-term health issues. Many contact sports have cultures that encourage athletes to continue playing despite injury and pain. However, studies suggest that these issues vary along racial and gender lines. A 1996 study on the subject notes that men are more likely than women to play through injury at personal cost, owing perhaps to stereotypes about masculinity (Nixon, 1996). The study also notes that Whites, are more likely to play through serious injury as well, due to greater trust in the predominantly White power structure in most sports (Nixon, 1996).

The amount of acute stress experienced by individual athletes, as well as the mechanisms they use to cope with stressors, can vary along racial and gender lines as well. A 2009 study on the subject notes that White athletes were more likely to cope with stress about performance by confiding in friends or family, where Black athletes were more likely to cope through self-assurance or religion (Anshel et al., 2009). This speaks once again to the additional resources and accommodating power structure provided to White athletes. The study also noted that "African American athletes were less comfortable with coach reprimands and other actions associated with an authoritative leadership style than were their Caucasian teammates," which again could be attributed to the fact that many more coaches—even those coaching Black athletes—are White than Black (Anshel et al., 2009).

The same study noted a similar trend in female athletes, who also tend disproportionately to have a male coach, reported more stressful coach/athlete relationships than their male counterparts and "perceive their male coach primarily as an authority figure" (Anshel et al., 2009). Additionally, the study found that female athletes tend to cope with stress more socially than men, increasing the necessity for positive athlete/coach relationships that female athletes often find lacking (Anshel et al., 2009).

In addition to the problems inherent in disparity within the structure of most athletic organizations, non-White and non-male athletes experience additional discrimination from the outside in the form of social abuse. Social media has changed many aspects of modern society, and sports is no exception. As it is to many, social media is a double-edged sword to many athletes, allowing them greater interaction with fans who can be anywhere from actively supportive to criminally abusive.

A 2019 study published in the *International Journal of Sport and Exercise Psychology* examined fan responses on social media when professional athletes violate norms. The study notes a baseline tendency for fans on social media to "send harmful comments of a sexual, physical, emotional, or discriminatory nature directly to athletes" even when they have not necessarily violated any societal norms. It also notes an increase in "dispute between athletes" on social media (MacPherson & Kerr, 2019).

The study concludes ultimately that while athletes face abuse on social media for a variety of reasons, the most common cause for an uptick in abuse toward a particular athlete is a social norm violation, followed by a legal violation, and lastly an athletic violation (in other words, a blunder on the field/court/rink/etc.) (MacPherson & Kerr, 2019). The study also notes that undue or inappropriate support on social media can do as much harm as abuse, referencing instances where athletes who have committed serious social or legal violations are excused by fans so long as they maintain their level of performance. An example is one social media post that said of a professional hockey player accused of rape: "He may be a rapist but he's a f****** beast" (MacPherson & Kerr, 2019).

While all athletes are susceptible to abuse at the hands of fans on social media, women and non-White athletes are particularly vulnerable to racist and sexist abuse. Perhaps the most succinct example is the case of aforementioned tennis star Serena Williams. A 2018 study into abuse of Williams on Twitter and Facebook during and following her participation in the 2015 Wimbledon Championships notes that Serena makes a good study case because of her "intersectionality," term used to describe someone who is vulnerable to multiple types of oppression due to membership in more than one oppressed group.

The paper concludes that social media provides a physical and perceived social "distance" between abuser and athlete, allowing the abuser to feel comfortable making comments and threats that they would not be comfortable making in person (Litchfield et al., 2018). Magnifying this effect is the fact that "Those who allot abuse in online spaces are often safe in the knowledge that their behavior has no consequence, at least legally" (Litchfield et al., 2018). The authors of the study argue that while sexism, racism, and stereotypes are not exclusive to social media by any means, the unregulated freedom of communication between any fan with an internet connection and world-famous athletes provides a fertile breeding ground (and public arena) for hate speech and abuse.

SUMMARY

Like many aspects of society, sports and athletics have come a long way in recent centuries and even recent decades in terms of equality and acceptance. Sports that once prohibited the participation of non-White people are often dominated by their presence. Sports from which women were once largely prohibited now feature professional or semi-professional leagues to showcase female athletes, and sports where women have long participated now feature and compensate women at an equal level to male participants.

However, like the many other aspects of society that have improved in recent times, sport still has a long way to go in providing equal opportunity, safety, and compensation for non-male and non-White athletes. While women and non-White people are more likely than ever to participate in sports or other athletics at the high-school, collegiate, and professional levels, the power structure of many of these sports remains inherently racist and sexist, with White males populating the vast majority of positions of power. In the NFL, for example, well over half of the athletes are non-White and many of them are Black. However, only four coaches are non-White and neither of two non-White team owners in the league are Black (Lapchick, 2019). While the athletes themselves do make more money than they used to, White owners still take the vast majority of the profit from the revenue their athleticism garners.

The increase of social connectivity in today's world, while it has its advantages, also provides a platform for athletes to receive additional abuse from fans. While this can affect all athletes, many observers feel comfortable espousing racist and sexist views on social media that they may not have previously been comfortable espousing or even admitting in public in previous years.

While many sports fans see sports as an escape from life, nothing could be further from the truth. Sports often reflect the changes taking place in society and culture. Sporting organizations are an example of myriad institutions that are still structured on discrimination. If we hope to dismantle the racism and sexism inherent in sports, we must work to change all of society. Then sports will undoubtedly reflect that change.

DISCUSSION QUESTIONS

1. What role does sexism play in sport?
2. How can sexism be solved?
3. How do gender stereotypes affect sports?

4. Give two examples of racism in sport that coaches can address.
5. How does racism affect participation? Where does racial disparity exist in sport?

REFERENCES

Anshel, M. H., Sutarso, T., & Jubenville, C. (2009). Racial and gender differences on sources of acute stress and coping type among competitive athletes. *The Journal of Social Psychology, 149*(2), 159–178. doi:10.3200/socp.149.2.159-178

Beamon, K. (2014). Racism and stereotyping on campus: Experiences of African American male student-athletes. *The Journal of Negro Education, 83*(2), 121. doi:10.7709/jnegroeducation.83.2.0121

Bodo, P. (2018, September). Follow the money: How the pay gap in Grand Slam tennis finally closed. *ESPN.com.*

Borish, L., & Gems, G. (2000). Ethnicity, gender, and sport in diverse historical contexts. *Journal of Sport History, 27*(3), 377–381.

Correia, M., Rosado, A., Serpa, S., & Ferreira, V. (2017). Fear of failure in athletes: Gender, age and type of sport differences. *Iberoamerican Journal of Psychology of Exercise and Sports, 12*(2), 185–193.

Hoberman, J. M. (1997). *Darwin's athletes: How sport has damaged Black America and preserved the myth of race.* Houghton Mifflin.

Lapchick, R. (2019, October). The NFL racial and gender report card. *ESPN.com.*

Litchfield, C., Kavanagh, E., Osborne, J., & Jones, I. (2018). Social media and the politics of gender, race and identity: The case of Serena Williams. *European Journal for Sport and Society, 15*(2), 154–170. Doi:10.1080/16138171.2018.1452870

MacPherson, E., & Kerr, G. (2019). Sport fans' responses on social media to professional athletes' norm violations. *International Journal of Sport and Exercise Psychology,* 1–18. doi:10.1080/1612197x.2019.1623283

National Collegiate Athletics Association. (2021). *Title IX frequently asked questions.* NCAA.org

National Women's Hockey League. (2021). *About the NWHL.* NWHL.zone/about-us

Nixon, H. (1996). Explaining pain and injury attitudes and experiences in sport in terms of gender, race, and sports status factors. *Journal of Sport and Social Issues, 20*(1), 33–44. doi:10.1177/019372396020001004

USWFL Football League. (n.d.). Home [Facebook Page]. *Facebook.* https://www.facebook.com/USWFL/about/?ref=page_internal

Women's National Basketball Association. (2021). *History.* WNBA.com

Challenges Experienced by Athletes

INTRODUCTION

The COVID-19 pandemic has caused not only environments of fear but also forced individuals and a nation to take a step back to consider how the future will change in light of current changes. The COVID-19 virus had spread throughout the world by December 2019, and by March 2020 the country had moved to full social distancing, mask wearing, and using the internet as a means of conducting business. March 2020 will be recorded historically as the period of change for American lifestyles. This shift impacted every aspect of American life, including America's favorite pastime—sports. As these changes are realized, this chapter presents a list of challenges experienced by athletes—not an exhaustive list, but instead a beginning list for students to discuss and add to strategies for overcoming the challenges.

MENTAL GAME CHALLENGES

During COVID-19, U.S. athletes experienced mental challenges unlike those ever seen in the history of American sports. The impact of these changes has yet to be realized, as the future is uncertain for many of these athletes. Mental health and physical health are equally important for the athlete. However, many professional and collegiate athletes are experiencing negative mental health issues as a result of their world being abruptly interrupted by the pandemic. The March 2020 decision to cancel the Olympic Games in Japan reinforced the need to adhere to the Centers for Disease Control and Prevention COVID-19 protocols (e.g., mask, gloves, social distancing). The 2020 Olympic Games were rescheduled to begin July 23, 2021, and end August 8, 2021, however, limited spectators were allowed. The fear and frustration impacted athlete's performances before, during, and after the Games.

Many athletes were affected emotionally as they attempted to train in an environment with a highly contagious virus inflicting fatal respiratory symptoms. Athletes experienced high levels of anxiety wondering whether the vaccine would protect them or whether their career would be over if infected by the virus. Anger also emerged due to feelings that professional athletes should be given priority with vaccines (Pound et al., 2021). The inequality of accessing vaccines even surfaced among the athletic community. There are debates as to whether the IOC/Pfizer deal was another political decision to ensure that all Olympian athletes received the Pfizer vaccine while underserved populations were more in need of the vaccine (Pound et al., 2021). This collaborative deal between the International Olympic Committee and the Pfizer company could also be considered as preempting some nation's mandates regarding who should be given the vaccine immediately because all nations do not have the same policies regarding the COVID-19 virus vaccine. For example, all athletes participating in the Olympic Games needed to have COVID-19 vaccinations, while Africa only administered 2% of the vaccinations (Moniuszko, 2021).

Olympians must be concerned about remaining healthy during this pandemic. Their mental health is a major concern. For example, the American gymnast Simone Biles revealed that mental health was her priority and that she was meeting with her psychologists weekly (Moniuszko, 2021).

Although the general public has been dealing with mental health issues since the pandemic began, athletes have experienced more pressures because they have to be concerned not only about the lack of or limited performance but also the impact on the future. Games were cancelled and stadiums were closed. Athletes isolated from the general public and games between teams occurred in the bubble. The bubble is the artificial environment designed for sports teams to play in isolation. The NBA bubble was the ESPN Worldwide Sports Complex that is located in Orlando, Florida (Medina, 2020). Once players were able to engage in their sports games, the isolation from fans, families, and communities could lead to depression or sleep disorders (Frank, 2020).

Seldom do fans of athletes consider the possibility that many athletes are fragile based on fear of failure and social approval. Athletes do not fear the virus, but they fear an inability to either return to past performance functioning levels or excel to a higher level of functioning. This ability can be interpreted as low self-confidence. In the sports arena, self-confidence is the ability to win games regardless of the situation (Andreato et al., 2020). Therefore, athletes must remember to continue their external conditioning and training. But how is this to become reality?

PHYSICAL CHALLENGES

During the pandemic, athletes have had to demonstrate that they can function autonomously by continuing to engage in daily conditioning and training. Many athletes used their daily conditioning as a means of stress reduction. Some athletes, however, do not use common sense to maintain career excellence, which Stambulova et al. (2020) describe as sustainability—a long, successful, and healthy career based on support from family, friends, teammates, and coaches. Prior to the pandemic, coaches and other team staff made sure that athletes were conditioning, training, and keeping dietary habits in sync with their assigned play positions. Sanctions were imposed if athletes did not adhere to the guidelines provided. However, during the pandemic years (2020–2021), athletes had to rely on themselves. Isolation can cause poor dietary habits resulting from anxiety and impulse and adverse behaviors such as drug abuse and detraining (Andreato et al., 2020). Detraining is the reduction or elimination of the rigorous training maneuvers that are mandatory in the training process to become an athlete. Just as isolation can cause detraining, detraining can also cause isolation. The athletes may not remain active physically, which and can cause harm by interfering with their emotional well-being. Isolation and confinement can also lead to numerous physical challenges for an athlete, such as muscle strength decline, increase in body fat, and less flexibility.

Some athletes who have been infected with the virus struggle to recover and obtain their original form. One such athlete is Jayson Tatum, NBA star of the Boston Celtics, who tested positive for the virus on January 9, 2020, and states that he still has difficulty simply running up and down the court. The majority of his time is now spent on rotation (Umeri, 2021).

Even though the vaccines are a health precaution there are still many unknow entities about the COVID-19 virus. It has been beneficial with reducing the number of infections however, the long-term effects are not known, which continues to cause fear and frustration among athletes as they press hard now in an uncertain future. Some countries such as Russia and China administered vaccines prior to third phase of the clinical trials (Gavi, 2020). The aftereffects are currently being studied. In the United States, the Johnson & Johnson/Janssen COVID-19 vaccine was administered with only 66% effectiveness in clinical trials. Yet the vaccine was one of the three administered in America. According to researchers in the Mayo Clinic (2020), there are four phases of human clinical trials: Phase 1: Test for safety (e.g., side effects); phase 2: Investigate efficacy on large group; phase 3: Test larger groups; and Phase 4: National regulatory approval (Gavi, 2020). The clinical trials started in summer 2020 in the United States. Typically clinical trials take approximately 2 years for FDA approval, but COVID-19 vaccines were approved in 6 months. The three approved vaccines delineated by the Mayo Clinic are as follows:

- Pfizer BioNTech COVID-19 vaccine with data suggesting a 95% effectiveness for the prevention of COVID-19 for ages 16 and older. Two injections are required, taken 21 days apart. Administered during phase 3 of clinical trials. The U.K. was the first country to approve Pfizer/Biontech, a German developed vaccine.
- Moderna COVID-19 Vaccine was developed in collaboration with the National Institute of Allergies and Infectious Diseases (NIAID) and the National Institutes of Health (NIH) in Cambridge, Massachusetts. The vaccine has a 94% effectiveness for prevention of serious effects from the virus in individuals 18 and older. It requires two injections, 28 days apart.
- Johnson & Johnson/Janssen COVID-19 Vaccine has more controversy than the Pfizer or Moderna. Although it requires only one injection, there was a pause placed on this vaccine due to possible blood clotting (Balzer, 2021). However, the vaccine was continued due to rationalizing that the blood clotting was less harmful than potential death from the virus. In the fourth clinical trials phase, the vaccine is still used in the United States and the Netherlands after the pause ended on April 26, 2021.

Although these vaccines have been distributed throughout the United States, the CDC continues to suggest wearing masks and practicing social distancing if the vaccine has not been administered. Most athletes have received their vaccine. However, the future with the virus remains uncertain.

WHAT ABOUT COLLEGIATE ATHLETES?

College athletes have suffered similar experiences of isolation, frustration, anger, and fear as professional athletes. However, a major difference is academics and extremely limited financial assistance. According to Kissinger and Miller (2009), student athletes generally face four distinctive challenges: balancing athletics and academics; balancing social activities with athletic responsibilities; balancing athletic success or lack of success; and balancing physical and mental health with continued competitiveness. Additionally, they may be challenged by trans athletic inclusions and the technological or digital world.

Balancing Athletics and Academics

Student athletes should focus on athletes as well as their academic schedule, and universities suggest that there is an equal focus on both. However, in too many instances this portrayal is false, with the focus on athletics. The rigor of the athlete's training schedules often clashes with scheduled classes or leaves them so exhausted from training sessions that they sit in the classroom in a lethargic state with limited or no cognitive responses to class interactions. Too often athletic students are unprepared with class assignments or they are unable to articulate in class the gist of the completed assigned work. Jayakumar and Comeaux (2016) revealed that there is inadequate organizational support for the dual role of higher education athletes, which leads to an unsuccessful academic experience. The term *cover-up* is used to describe the limited or lack of academic success for most athletes. In an academic environment where the expectations should be focused on academics, athletes face the challenge of attempting to navigate an unrealistic balancing act (Jayakumar & Comeaux, 2016). Many athletes, especially those from disadvantaged communities, need tutors who can assist them with learning the basics (reading, writing, and math) that were not mastered in high school. Yet there is often limited time with tutors, or no time at all for assistance with their classwork. Stories and jokes are often heard about athletes who have tutors completing their classwork or about athletic advisors selecting "easy" class schedules for athletes.

What is seldom discussed is the pain that athletes experience when they desperately want to receive an education. Many want to graduate with knowledge—and not simply graduate. These athletes struggle with the stereotypes, the jokes, and the images of "dumb athlete." The blame is placed on the athlete when the blame really lies with the degree-granting college or university. Just as athletes receive penalties for foul play on the field or court, higher education organizations should receive penalties for not graduating athletes who have poured their souls into bringing money into the organization, and for granting unearned degrees to athletes who leave the organization still unable to read, write, or speak simple sentences. If higher education receives negative monetary sanctions, more athletes will graduate from programs and will be able to display an ability to read and write at a college level, which is especially true for African American male athletes (Outlaw, 2019). There is the suggestion that this should be considered risky health behavior, requiring intervention strategies to increase success rates, change attitudes, and increase levels of knowledge and academic skills (McDougle & Capers, 2012).

Balancing Social Activities With Athletic Responsibilities

Athletic departments function autonomously within higher education organizations. The location is typically away from the main campus or, if on main campus, the proximity is a hub spaciously located away from other buildings and surrounded by a stadium, track field, and gymnasium. All resources (medical staff and equipment, workout rooms, tutors, advisors, coaches, trainers, lockers, lecture rooms, and dorms) are within the athletic hub. This produces challenges for athletes who may not have experienced an academic struggle in high school or college by limiting their external career perspectives.

The priority is on their athleticism, and therefore exposure to career options after athletics is limited due to their isolation by athletic departments. This is especially the case for African American athletes in predominately White colleges and universities who may not have exposure during their academic years to a nonathletic professional who looks like them (McDougle & Capers, 2012). Many of these athletes are not exposed to career choice possibilities. Although some institutions of higher education develop program initiatives to increase the numbers of underrepresented minority students of color, these programs seldom include student athlete recruits due to athletic schedules. Therefore, these academically talented student athletes are also academically underserved by the higher education organization. For example, Ohio State University's medical camp program was designed to increase the number of minorities entering medical school programs but is not realistic for athletes at the school because of their athletic schedules. Thus, athletes who are overachievers and those who may be underachieving academically are not receiving the necessary guidance to enter nonathletic careers after their college career.

Balancing Athletic Success or Lack of Success

Playing sports is an exciting dream for many collegiate athletes. This dream may be enforced by the love of sports, the desire to help the family, a wish to become famous, or the urge to win. Professional sports is the gateway to accomplishing their dream, but many hopes and dreams are shattered by the reality that only 2% of NCAA collegiate athletes are able to enter professional sports (Carter, 2019). This reality alone should force institutions of higher education to also focus on careers for their athletes. These athletes dedicate three or more years of loyalty to their sport with very limited or no concern for their personal career passion after the sport. For some, the timeline is shortened by injuries that eliminate their usefulness to the sport, and they are left isolated from the athletic hub, and, in some instances, engulfed with depression and uncertainties. The challenge for these athletes is figuring out what to do next.

Balancing Physical and Mental Health With Continued Competitiveness

The transition from collegiate athlete to life after the sport can be a devasting factor in the lives of many athletes. This is due to the fact that many have not focused on post-sports planning. This dilemma becomes even more traumatic for athletes who experience injuries and cannot return to the game. They experience a sense of shame, guilt, and numerous losses (team, coach, fans, and their identity). Some may indulge in painkiller medications, while others may wander in hopelessness, attempting to discover remedies, and still others who are unable to handle the loss and may engage in illegal substances as a means of coping. The tragedy is that these athletes are not provided with resources to assist them in their time(s) of need.

Most institutions of higher education (especially NCAA division institutions) have mental health units on campus to assist students with emotional and psychological needs during their academic years. However, these units are often not utilized by athletes because they are external units "outside" of the athletic department. Also, many collegiate athletes do not want the stigma of identification with emotional or psychological issues. Therefore, they suffer in silence. The University of Michigan has provided a model for sports afterlife with their program designed specifically to assist their collegiate athletes begin to consider life after the sport.

A strong advocate for the program is Jeff Porter, a former 2007 NCAA champion in hurdles and a former Olympian representing the U.S. team in hurdles. He discovered life after athletics by earning his doctorate in 2017, and he currently serves as chair of the Athletes Advisory Committee for U.S. Track and Field (USATF) and as a member of its board of directors. Porter suggests the need for higher education athletic programs to become more inclusive of focus on academic and career goals (Leef, 2021). He promotes assisting athletes to find their passions outside sports and mentoring as key features to relieve some of their "after sports" stressors. His suggestion to begin these discussions early as an essential tool to athletic success is reasonable. However, higher educational organizations have a tendency to "talk the talk but not walk the walk" in areas where minorities are the concern (Outlaw, 2019). Thus, the need is to incorporate an embedded program component within the athletic department's programing. It would include a clinical component inclusive of provisions for counseling, mentoring, identifying career goals, discovering self-identity, and discussing accounting and marketing and coping strategies for stress reduction. This sports clinical component (Outlaw, 2019) can relieve and resolve many of the issues that collegiate and professional athletes constantly struggle with that too often lead to devastating outcomes of harm to either self or others. The sports clinic embedded within the athletic department can serve as a holistic entity that will allow athletes to balance the challenges of life after sports in a nonjudgmental and effective environment. This clinic can also provide therapeutic discussions to address unresolved family issues and make life understandable. Then athletes will be armed with effective strategies and mentors to assist them during and after they leave the sport.

CHALLENGES OF TRANS ATHLETES

Trans athletes experience even more challenges as they struggle to exist in an environment of contradictions in the U.S., where there are verbal outcries against discriminatory practices and written laws to protect individual rights, yet overt actions taken against individuals simply because they are different. Actions taken against transgendered athletes in sports are taken in the name of "fairness" where the verbal and written actions suggest that there is an unfair advantage in having a biological male who has transitioned to female competing in a sport against biological female athletes. However, the argument of fairness is seldom mentioned in situations of biological females who have transitioned to male and choose to compete against biological male athletes. For example, there was great media coverage on Quinn, a Canadian Olympic soccer athlete who helped to win the gold in the Tokyo games. Quinn, who was biologically assigned as a female at birth, identified as a nonbinary athlete (not male or female). Historical records will log Quinn as the first transgender to win an Olympic gold medal. Laurel Hubbard, from New Zealand, will be listed as the first transgender competitor in individual sports in the Olympics weightlifting category. Although considered a medalist competitor, Hubbard did not win a medal (Boren, 2021).

The Olympic Committee allowed trans athletes to participate in Olympic Games in 2004, and the numbers have been increasing since that time. Although 2021 marked the historical underpinnings for trans athletes with 163 LGBTQ+ athletes participating in the Olympic Games (three times more than in the 2016 Rio games), it is important to take a moment to understand some of the challenges experienced by trans individuals. Knowledge reduces the likelihood of fears based on unknown information about genders and gender roles.

The psychologist John Money is credited with coining the term *gender* in 1955, which he described as a basic human characteristic (Goldie, 2014). Although Money is described as a sexologist who advocated for sexual liberation, his sexual reassignment experimentation with David Reimer caused a great deal of controversy based on Reimer's account of the experimentation. Reimer was born biologically a male. However, due to phimosis (failure of the penis foreskin to retract) he underwent circumcision, and his penis was damaged during the procedure beyond functioning ability. John Money recommended sexual reassignment (Gaetano, 2017). Reimer's testes and damaged penis were removed, and David was raised as a girl from infancy, receiving estrogen in his adolescent years (Giese & Wodskou, 2015). David Reimer is considered the first documented case of sex reassignment. However, he was not informed that he was originally a male, and after the discovery while in his 20s, he attempted suicide on two different occasions. At the age of 38, he was successful in his attempt, ending his life with a firearm (Gaetano, 2017). He had suffered from depression all of his adult life (Giese & Wodskou, 2015).

John Money's contribution to gender identity and gender roles provide a foundation for discussions related to sexual identity and gender identity as our understanding of gender continues to suggest the need for change and the need to focus on marketing as a means of intensifying change (McIntyre, 2018). For example, the concept of cis (cisgender) was recently added to the Oxford dictionary in 2015, and it relates specifically to gender as opposed to sexuality (McIntyre, 2018). It is the sex that is assigned at birth, and that is the sex used for identification. When discussing transgender individuals, it is significant to distinguish the difference between gender and sexuality. Transgender is used to identify individuals who identify their gender as different than their assigned sex (when they were born) (Rivera, 2021). The individual chooses to decide whether they are male or female or nonbinary (gender identity is neither male nor female) or agender (without a particular gender).

The International Olympic Committee has officially recognized transgender athletes as official Olympic Game participants since 2004 (Boren, 2021); however, the United States continues to struggle with allowing transgender student athletes to perform in sports based on their gender choice. Idaho was the first state to pass legislation against transgender athletes participating in school and college sports (Cancian, 2021). House Bill 500 prevented birth gender assigned athletes from participating in sports that differed from the gender assigned at birth (Rivera, 2021). Although the bill was not implemented because of a federal court's ruling of discrimination against transgendered individuals, other states began to introduce similar bills to exclude transgender youth from participating in sports. Although the states are citing disadvantage of competition, researcher Harper (2015) found that transgender distant runners were not more competitive as women than as men. Harper's studies suggests that transgender athletes perform at the same level as cisgender athletes, and it was Harper who assisted with writing the International Olympic Committee's transgender policy (Hollingsworth, 2021).

President Biden has attempted to intervene with the signing of Executive Order 13988, prohibiting discrimination in school sports based on gender identity and not based on gender assignment at birth (Cancian, 2021). This Executive Order, along with the Department of Justice's mandate to enforce sexual antidiscrimination laws that protect gender identity under Title IX (Sharrow, 2021) and NCAA's indication that discrimination against transgender athletes is not an acceptable practice, may deter some states from taking actions. However, although these nondiscriminatory protections are beginning safeguards, the United States will continue to experience court battles and covert and overt discrimination against transgender athletes. Although not representing all transgender women, Martina Navratilova (tennis), Sharron Davies (swimming), Kelly Holmes and Paula Radcliffe (marathon) shared publicly their thoughts about unfairness of trans women who compete in women's elite sports: (a) rules endorsed by International Olympic Committee are problematic; (b) unfairness and advantage of performance are reasons to not allow them to compete; and (c) requirement of allyship requires more from women athletes than can reasonably be expected (Teetzel, 2020).

State laws vary regarding eligibility requirements for transgender athletes. Many states continue to argue the unfairness of transgender participation in sports based on testosterone levels, even though current peer-reviewed science suggests that athletes' sports achievements are the result of many different factors and such features as hormones and chromosomes should not be the deciding factor for successful performance (Sharrow, 2021). The lack of conclusive data on the impact of transgender athletes on sports performance versus cisgender athletes' sports performance remains unclear. Best practice medical care suggests that transgender youth athletes should be supported in an effort to deter life-threatening circumstances (Stahl, 2021) because many of these youth experience trauma from external sources (e.g., peers, teachers, and sports fans and in some instances, family members). As a result, they seem to be more prone to depression, self-harm, low self-esteem, and suicidal tendencies (Stahl, 2021). Research by Toomey et al. (2018) provides shocking statistics on the suicide rates among transgender adolescents. Female to male adolescents reported the highest attempted suicide rate of any gender identity category at 50.8%. This group was followed by the binary gender category at 41.8%, with male to female adolescents at 29.9% from a sample size of $N = 120,617$ in adolescents aged 11–19 years. This study revealed that suicidal behaviors (including either planning or attempting suicide) was higher in trans adolescents than in cisgender adolescents.

It is extremely important for families to support their adolescents who may be experiencing gender identity changes, especially if the adolescent is engaged in sports. Family support can provide the emotional and psychological support that may be missing in interactions with peers and other external micro and macro systems. Stahl (2021) suggests that family support can reduce suicidal thoughts within trans adolescents by 52% and decrease suicide attempts by 48% as well. Although many transgender adolescents do not participate in sports primarily because the sports infrastructure does not support them, according to Hollingsworth (2021), there is still the need to focus on efforts to ensure that those trans adolescents who are participating in sports are not mistreated with transphobic attitudes or recipients of discriminatory practices.

Prior to Title IX, interscholastic sports were designed primarily for males (Sharrow, 2021) with little thought given to females and no thought given to transgender athletes. Sports teams were segregated male and female teams. Currently there is public awareness that transgender athletes are increasing in numbers, and therefore, athletic committees, owners, and teams will have to implement policies that are inclusive of those with various gender identities. Not only are the systemic challenges in need of modifications at the macro level, but micro level challenges directed at specific trans individuals will also need to be addressed as many of these athletes experience personal harassment, bullying, exclusion from social activities, and physical assaults.

Numerous challenges are faced by athletes, whether cisgender or LGBTQ, in local, national, and international sports, whether college athlete, professional, or Olympian, they all must overcome similar challenges. These challenges can be dichotomized into two distinct categories: performance expectations and social development. Performance expectations focus on the sport as the priority. Coaches consider athletic performance above all other factors (including injuries). If a player is hurt on the field, the question is whether the athlete can continue to complete in the game and not what the injury is or how the athlete is affected. Social development encompasses the Socratic perspective of knowing thyself, yet many athletes are unclear about anything that does not involve sports. Even though college is typically a place to "find yourself" and discover your passion, many athletes do not discover their passion, and when they leave the game, they are left to figure out what they can do other than sports. This awakening is at times cruel because their social interactions are limited to teammates; there is limited time for family or friends due to the rigorous schedule (e.g., training, games, and practices). Thus, their social skills may also need adjustment because collegiate experiences may have held limited social interactions. The athletes who graduate discover that life after sport is a lonely place. Therapeutic intervention may prove beneficial; however, they must discard the previous negative thinking regarding therapeutic intervention and seek effective coping strategies that can lead to success after leaving the sport.

Technological Challenges Facing Sports Industry

Technology has "upped" the sports game with the need to remain aware of technological advances that impact sports. Teams are forced to constantly update their websites (Twitter feeds, Facebook) to keep fans following them. Attendance at games has been primarily via virtual viewing during the pandemic. The virtual aspect of sports has advantages and disadvantages. Some advantages include increased numbers of viewers with more people watching the sports on cell phones or iPad, increased purchasers of season tickets who view their favorite sports team, increased knowledge about sports from fans, and increased contact and interactions with favorite athletes via Tweets/Facebook. Some disadvantages include limited or no use of million-dollar stadiums, which reduces the revenue for the city (among restaurants, hotels, and retail stores), makes players unable to receive the stimulation or motivation from fans during play, and decreases of social game interactions among fans. The jury is still out discovering whether esports is an advantage or disadvantage.

Esports or electronic sports are sports games that are organized by teams or players who play against each other for prizes and the title of "best in the world," since these events are worldwide events This gaming event has become nationally recognized, and collegiate and professional sports have entered the esports gaming arena. This organized video gaming competition is watched by over 165 million of people from North American, China, and South Korea who are constant viewers of the esports games (Willingham, 2018). In 2021, esports were valued at over one billion dollars in the global market (Willings, 2021).

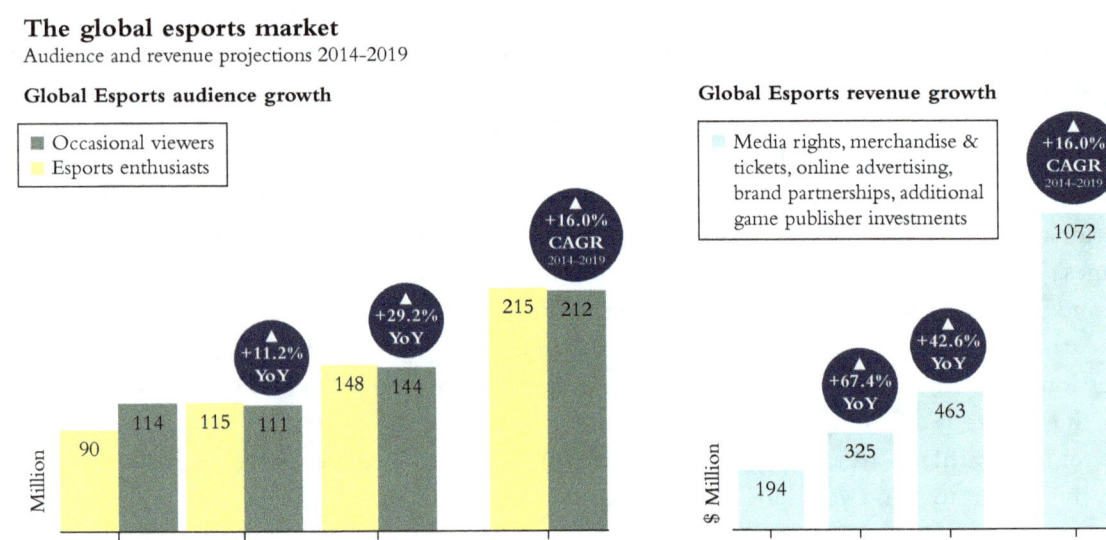

FIGURE 6.1   *The Global eSports Market*

Adair (n.d.) suggests that the winner of the first esports game was in 1972, with the winner receiving a *Rolling Stone* magazine subscription as the prize. However, esports games had their worldwide notice in the 1990s as a causal hobby that reached "gold mine" heights. Major television networks such as TBS, ESPN, and SYFY are among those broadcasting esports games. Adair (n.d.) further provides a listing of the most popular esports games (such as Legends of Leagues, Fortnite, and DOTA2) based on monetary prizes and number of fans. He states that it is difficult to identify the best esports teams due to the diverse nature of the gaming events where some individual participants can compete in different esports or as an individual player. More viewers are watching esports games than the traditional sports games, which creates a need for further exploration by sports owners and coaches. From a *Rolling Stones* subscription to winning millions of dollars, the esports games have become the sports to watch—the sports that may replace traditional sports games.

Zhang et al. (2018) suggest the need for researchers to investigate the challenges that future virtual sports games will have on the sports industry. They strongly encourage the need to advance theoretical perspectives and solutions around sports and their economic and marketing effects. There is limited research done on esports gaming (Rogers et al., 2020), and the call to action is to motivate and fund more research in this area of specialty. With the increasing popularity of competitive esports games, there is also an increase in unregulated gaming subculture using digital currency to place bets in esporting events (Greer et al., 2019).

Digital currency is termed *cryptocurrency* and is a form of technological monetary exchange. It is equivalent to the U.S. dollar, but in digital coins, with Bitcoin currently being the best-known cryptocurrency supported by blockchain technology (Delfabbro et al., 2021). Cryptocurrency is widely accepted by mainstream audiences because of its easy accessibility, 24-hour scope of time, social networking, and increased use by less experienced investors.

TABLE 6.1 Analysis of Crypto-Wagering Sites

Sportsbook	Location	Sports Branding	Unique Daily Visitors	Top-level Domain	Server Location	SBR Rating	Online Since	Accept Aust Bets?
Bookmaker	Costa Rica	Basketball, ice hockey, gridiron, baseball, soccer	5,950	.eu	Costa Rica	A+	2000	Yes
5Dimes	Costa Rica	None	21,950	.eu	USA	A+	2000	Yes
BetOnline	Panama	Basketball, gridiron	13,100	.ag	Panama	A+	2001	Yes
Bovada	—	Basketball, ice hockey, basketball	51,000	.lv	Canada	A+	2011	—
Heritage sports	Costa Rica	Gridiron	1,650	.eu	Costa Rica	A+	2001	Yes
BetDSI	Costa Rica	Gridiron	7,600	.eu	USA	A	2001	Yes
SportsBetting	Panama	Gridiron	4,879	.ag	Panama	A	1998	Yes
JustBet	Panama	Gridiron	145	.cx	Costa Rica	A	2000	Yes
Intertops	Antigua	Gridiron	12,100	.eu	Antigua	A	1996	Yes
YouWager	Costa Rica	Gridiron	650	.eu	Costa Rica	A	1999	Yes
WagerWeb	Costa Rica	Gridiron	140	.ag	Costa Rica	B+	1999	Yes
GTbets	Curacao	Gridiron, horses	975	.eu	UK	B+	2011	Yes
Nitrogen sports	Costa Rica	Gridiron	8,050	.eu	USA	B+	2012	Yes
JazzSports	Costa Rica	Gridiron, horses	100	.ag	USA	B	2000	Yes
BetPhoenix	Costa Rica	Gridiron, basketball	500	.ag	USA	B	2006	Yes
Skybook	Costa Rica	Gridiron	15	.ag	USA	B	1998	Yes
BetMania	Costa Rica	Basketball	45	.ag	USA	B	2004	Yes
Anonibet	United Kingdom	None	170	.com	USA	C+	2011	Yes
BitcoinRush	—	Gridiron	1,050	.io	USA	C+	2013	Yes
HRWager	Costa Rica	Gridiron	150	.com	USA	C+	2012	Yes
Cloudbet	Montenegro	Gridiron, basketball, soccer	9,850	.com	USA	C+	2013	Yes
Betcoin	—	None	1,850	.com	USA	C+	2013	Yes
Sportsbet.io	Curacao	Soccer	2,000	.io	USA	C+	2016	Yes
MyBookie	Costa Rica	Gridiron	825	.ag	Canada	C	2014	Yes

(continued)

Chapter 6 Challenges Experienced by Athletes | 67

TABLE 6.1 Analysis of Crypto-Wagering Sites (Continued)

Sportsbook	Location	Sports Branding	Unique Daily Visitors	Top-level Domain	Server Location	SBR Rating	Online Since	Accept Aust Bets?
Bodog sportsbook	Antigua	Gridiron, ice hockey, basketball	6,850	.eu	Canada	A+	2003	–
Betcris	Costa Rica	Soccer	10,450	.com	Costa Rica	A+	2000	Yes
The Greek Sportsbook	Jamaica	Gridiron	800	.com	USA	A+	1998	Yes
Sportbet	Costa Rica	Gridiron, basketball, soccer, ice hockey	1,800	.com	USA	A	1997	Yes
Vietbet	Costa Rica	Gridiron	448	.eu	Costa Rica	A	2002	Yes
Galaxy Sport	Costa Rica	–	–	–	–	A	2014	Yes
IslandCasino	Costa Rica	Gridiron, soccer	632	.com	Costa Rica	A-	1997	Yes
BetAnySports	Costa Rica	Gridiron, baseball	390	.eu	Costa Rica	A-	2001	Yes
ChineseBookie	Costa Rica	Baseball	20	.eu	Netherlands	A-	2005	Yes
BetDNA	Costa Rica	–	–	–	–	D+	2012	Yes
BetOwi	Costa Rica	Gridiron	–	.com	Taiwan	D	2011	Yes
Sportsbook.com	Antigua	Gridiron	1,197	.com	Antigua	D-	2000	–

From: How can legislators protect sport from the integrity threat posed by cryptocurrencies? https://link.springer.com/article/10.1007/s40318-018-0132-0/tables/2

Sources: For Location, SBR Rating, Online Since, and Accepts Australian Bets, the relevant review page at Sportsbook Review, *Betting Sites*, https://www.sportsbookreview.com/betting-sites/; For Unique Daily Visitors and Server Location, by searching the relevant site at Hypestat, http://www.hypestat.com; For Branding and Top Level Domain, by visiting the sites.

Cryptocurrency is a digital currency used for virtual transactions that are not covered by a bank or other financial institution. The transactions are directly between the individuals (Akar & Akar, 2020). Naraine (2019) argues that cryptocurrency is beneficial to sports. There is an increase in individual participation and sports betting and technology offers an improved method of data management. The United States has a number of wager sites since 1997. The increased number of betting sites that use the bitcoin cryptocurrency has also caused a new set of challenges for policy makers and law enforcement as the anonymity offered in cryptocurrency wagers can hinder enforcements.

Esports gambling has increased to the point of predictions that it will revolutionize sports gambling transactions (Gainsbury & Blaszczynski, 2017) and present cause to focus on more research in the areas of gambling addiction treatment and egambling policies and laws. The world of sports will refocus on issues related to match-fixing, fraudulent ticket manufacturing, and equity viewing and participation. This is similar to the stock market, and everyone does not understand or participate in the stock market (Holzhauer, 2022). Although these may appear to be realistic goals with cryptocurrencies and Blockchain, the world of sports has not realized their importance. Discussions about these issues must begin now if we are to have a positive impact on the future of sports gambling because the digital coin is the future. Numerous challenges require consideration in esports: cryptocurrencies with limited or lack of regulatory infrastructure, the potential for increased criminal activity due to anonymity of participants, and security and private information issues.

SUMMARY

Athletes face numerous challenges daily, and it is at times difficult for the shouting fans to realize their impact on athletes. Fans can stimulate and motivate athletes to perform well, or fans can provide destructive attitudes and behaviors that can also impact athletic performance. Athletes are in need of a strong support system external to the athletic department but in collaboration with the athletic department. The major priority for the athletic department is to win games. Without exception, if an athlete cannot perform well, that athlete becomes an obsolete entity in the locker room and on the team. The challenge for the athlete becomes the question, what's next? What can I do or what do I want to do? Life becomes really scary because the athlete has never had to think about life after the sport. The athlete faces loss of identity, loss of skill, loss of fans, loss of feeling special, loss of teammates, loss of early morning workouts/training, and loss of structure—all losses that can cause emotional and psychological distress. Therefore, there is an urgent need to encourage more research into the athletic challenges identified in this chapter. To ignore these challenges is likened to coaches ignoring every aspect of their players and only focusing on their game performance.

DISCUSSION QUESTIONS

1. In a group, formulate strategies that can be used to overcome at least three challenges that you read about in this chapter.
2. Discuss your thoughts regarding a specific NCAA restriction.

3. Identify and describe a sports court case, and explain your thoughts regarding the court's decision on the case.
4. Using the internet, locate a Facebook, Twitter or team web page and provide an assessment. For example, consider how recently it has been updated, whether the information is current, and what should be different.
5. In a small group, discuss the issues related to social justice and trans sports athletes.
6. What are your thoughts about cryptocurrencies and the future related to gaming transactions?

REFERENCES

Adair, C. (n.d.). What is esports? History, top teams, revenues and risks [blog]. *Game Quitters*. https://gamequitters.com/what-is-esports/

Akar, S., & Akar, E. (2020). Is it a new tulip mania age: A comprehensive literature review beyond cryptocurrencies, bitcoin, and blockchain technology. *Journal of Information Technology Research, 13*(1), 24. doi: 10.4018/JITR.2020010104; https://www.igi-global.com/article/is-it-a-new-tulip-mania-age/240721

Andreato, L., Coimbra, D. R., & Andrade, A. (2020). Challenges to athletes during the home confinement caused by the COVID-19 pandemic. *Strength and Conditioning Journal*. https://www.ncbi.nlm.nih.gov/pmc/articles/PMC7219846/

Balzer, D. (2021). J & J COVID-19 vaccine pause ends. Mayo Foundation for Medical Education and Research. https://newsnetwork.mayoclinic.org/discussion/jj-covid-19-vaccine-pause-ends/

Boren, C. (2021, August 2). Canadian soccer player makes history as first openly trans athlete to medal in the Olympics. *The Washington Post*. https://www.washingtonpost.com/sports/olympics/2021/08/02/quinn-canada-soccer-transgender-athlete-olympics-medal/

Cancian, D. (2021, March 12). Transgender athletes are banned from sports in these states. *Newsweek*. https://www.newsweek.com/transgender-athletes-banned-sports-these-us-states-1575659

Carter, M. (2019, November 26). Leaving athletics can be "huge void" for former student-athletes. *Global Sport Matters*. Global Sport Institute, Arizona State University. https://globalsportmatters.com/culture/2019/11/26/leaving-athletics-can-be-huge-void-for-former-student-athletes/

Delfabbro, P., King, D. L., & Williams, J. (2021). The psychology of cryptocurrency trading: Risk and protective factors. *Journal of Behavioral Addictions, 10*(2), 201–207. https://akjournals.com/view/journals/2006/10/2/article-p201.xml?body=pdf-23898

Frank, A., Fatke, B., Frank, W., Förstl, H., & Hölzle, P. (2020). Depression, dependence and prices of the COVID-19-crisis. *Brain, Behavior, and Immunity, 87*. doi: 10.1016/j.bbi.2020.04.068

Gaetano, P. (2017). David Reimer and John Money gender reassignment controversy: The John/Joan case. *Embryo project encyclopedia*. http://embryo.asu.edu/handle/10776/13009; https://embryo.asu.edu/pages/david-reimer-and-john-money-gender-reassignment-controversy-johnjoan-case

Gainsbury, S. M., & Blaszczynski, A. (2017). How blockchain and cryptocurrency technology could revolutionize online gambling. *Gaming Law Review, 21*(7). https://doi.org/10.1089/glr2.2017.2174; https://www.liebertpub.com/doi/full/10.1089/glr2.2017.2174

Gavi. (2021, July 7). COVID-19 updates. The COVID-19 vaccine race. https://www.gavi.org/vaccineswork/covid-19-vaccine-race

Goldie, T. (2014). *The man who invented gender.* UBC Press.

Giese, R., & Wodskou, C. (2015, July 5). The story of John Money: Controversial sexologist grappled with the concept of gender. *CBC News.* https://www.cbc.ca/news/canada/the-story-of-john-money-controversial-sexologist-grappled-with-the-concept-of-gender-1.3137670

Greer, N., Rockloff, M., Browne, M., Hing, N., & King, D. L. (2019). Esports betting and skin gambling: A brief history. *Journal of Gambling Issues, 43.* https://jgi.camh.net/index.php/jgi/article/view/4059

Hollingsworth, J. (2021, July 4). A transgender weightlifter's Olympic dream has sparked an existential debate about what it means to be female. *CNN.* https://www.cnn.com/2021/07/03/sport/transgender-athletes-tokyo-olympics-intl-hnk-dst/index.html

Holzhauer, J. (2022). How sports betting and the stock market compare. *The Athletic.* https://theathletic.com/3554635/2022/09/01/sports-betting-and-financial-markets/

Jayakumar, U. M., & Comeaux, E. (2016). The cultural cover-up of college athletics: How organizational culture perpetuates an unrealistic and idealized balancing act. *The Journal of Higher Education, 87*(4), 488–515. doi: 10.1080/00221546.2016.11777411; https://www.tandfonline.com/doi/abs/10.1080/00221546.2016.11777411

Kissinger, D. B., & Miller, M. T. (2009). *College student-athletes.* Information Age Publishing Inc.

Leef, G. (2021). Recalling the great UNC sports scandal—How much has really changed. James G. Martin Center for Academic Renewal. https://www.jamesgmartin.center/2021/09/recalling-the-great-unc-sports-scandal-how-much-has-really-changed/

Mayo Clinic. (2021). COVID-19 vaccines: Get the facts. https://www.mayoclinic.org/diseases-conditions/coronavirus/in-depth/coronavirus-vaccine/art-20484859#:~:text=Janssen%2FJohnson%20%26%20Johnson%20COVID-19%20vaccine.&text=In%20clinical%20trials%2C%20this%20vaccine,least%2028%20days%20after%20vaccination

McDougle, L., & Capers, Q. (2012). Establishing priorities for student-athletes: Balancing academics and sports. *Spectrum: A Journal on Black Men, 1*(1), 71–77. https://doi.org/10.2979/spectrum.1.1.71

McIntyre, M. P. (2018). Gender by design: Performativity and consumer packaging. *Design and Culture, 10*(3), 337–358. doi: 10.1080/17547075.2018.1516437; https://www.tandfonline.com/doi/full/10.1080/17547075.2018.1516437

Medina, M. (2020, September 7). Challenges of isolated life in the bubble add to NBA players' playoff stress: "I just checked out." *USA Today.* https://www.usatoday.com/story/sports/nba/2020/09/07/nba-players-grapple-with-mental-health-inside-nba-bubble/5742849002/

Moniuszko, S. M. (2021, July 12). Simone Biles, Ginny Fuchs and more Olympians talk about prioritizing mental health. *USA Today.* https://www.usatoday.com/story/life/health-wellness/2021/07/12/olympics-simone-biles-talks-psychologist-ginny-fuchs-ocd/7934904002/

Naraine, M. (2019). The blockchain phenomenon: Conceptualizing decentralized networks and the value proposition to the sport industry. *International Journal of Sport Communication, 12*(3), 313–335. https://journals.humankinetics.com/view/journals/ijsc/12/3/article-p313.xml

Outlaw, K. R. (2019, December). *Exploring the challenges of elite African American male athletes at predominately White universities: Three descriptive case studies* (Doctoral dissertation, East Carolina University). http://hdl.handle.net/10342/7617

Pound, R. W., Grand'Maison, V., Robinson-Hill, L., & Lenskyj, H. J. (2021). The Saturday debate: Should Olympic athletes get priority to COVID-19 vaccines? *Toronto Star Newspaper.* https://www.thestar.com/

opinion/contributors/the-saturday-debate/2021/05/15/the-saturday-debate-should-olympic-athletes-get-priority-to-covid-19-vaccines.html

Rivera, A. (2021, May 11). A look at shifting trends in transgender athlete policies. *National Conference of State Legislatures.* https://www.ncsl.org/research/education/a-look-at-shifting-trends-in-transgender-athlete-policies-magazine2021.aspx

Rogers, R., Farquhar, L., & Mummert, J. (2020). Audience response to endemic and non-endemic sponsors of esports events. *International Journal of Sports Marketing and Sponsorship, 21*(3), 561–576. https://doi.org/10.1108/IJSMS-09-2019-0107

Sharrow, E. (2021). Five states ban transgender girls from girls' school sports. But segregating sports by sex hurts all girls. *The Washington Post.* https://www.washingtonpost.com/politics/2021/04/16/five-states-ban-transgender-girls-girls-school-sports-segregating-sports-by-sex-hurts-all-girls/

Stahl, S. (2021, March 14). Mythbuster: Debunking anti-transgender messages. *Freedom for All Americans Education Fund.* https://freedomforallamericans.org/mythbuster-debunking-anti-transgender-messages/?gclid=EAIaIQobChMIvuf4oIfl8QIVCnNvBB0NAwEPEAAYASAAEgLE0fD_BwE

Stambulova, N. B., Schinke, R. J., Lavallee, D., & Wylleman, P. (2020). The COVID-19 pandemic and Olympic/Paralympic athletes' developmental challenges and possibilities in times of a global crisis-transition. *International Journal of Sport and Exercise Psychology, 20*(1), 92–101. doi: 10.1080/1612197X.2020.1810865

Teetzel, S. (2020). Allyship in elite women's sport. *Sport, Ethics and Philosophy, 14*(4), 432–448. doi: 10.1080/17511321.2020.1775691; https://www.tandfonline.com/doi/abs/10.1080/17511321.2020.1775691

Toomey, R. B., Syvertsen, A. K., & Shramko, M. (2018). Transgender adolescent suicide behavior. *Pediatrics, 142*(4). doi: 10.1542/peds.2017-4218; https://pediatrics.aappublications.org/content/142/4/e20174218

Umeri, S. (2021, March 3). How elite athletes have struggled with the long-term effects of COVID. *SB Nation.* https://www.sbnation.com/nba/2021/3/3/22292213/athletes-covid-recovery-stories-jayson-tatum-mo-bamba-asia-durr

Willingham, A. J. (2018, August 27). What is esports? A look at an explosive billion dollar industry. *CNN.* https://www.cnn.com/2018/08/27/us/esports-what-is-video-game-professional-league-madden-trnd/index.html

Willings, A. (2021, October 11). What is esports and why is it a big deal? *Pocket-lint.* https://www.pocket-lint.com/games/news/145890-what-is-esports-professional-gaming-explained

IMAGE CREDIT

Fig. 6.1: Source: https://www.cnn.com/2018/08/27/us/esports-what-is-video-game-professional-league-madden-trnd/index.html.

NCAA Response to Drug Use Among Collegiate Athletes

INTRODUCTION

The National Collegiate Athletic Association (NCAA) is a member-led organization dedicated to the well-being and lifelong success of college athletes at 1,098 colleges and universities (NCAA, 2021). While the NCAA has many priorities, including academics and fairness, the area of well-being and safety in college sports is of paramount importance. Part of well-being and safety is a focus on substance abuse, including alcohol use and illicit substance abuse. In 1985, the NCAA conducted its initial "National Study of Substance Use Habits of College Student-Athletes" and in 1986, the NCAA began to administer drug tests for banned drugs (National Collegiate Athletic Association, 2012). Since that first report, additional studies have been completed with updates to improve the feedback and reflect the changes of society, as well as the culture where student athletes live, work, and play. This chapter examines substance abuse among NCAA student athletes.

The NCAA requires mandatory drug testing in addition to any member schools' drug testing policies. The NCAA examines "the use and abuse habits of college student-athletes every four years" (Green et al., 2001, p. 51). Under the NCAA rules, all Division I and Division II student athletes are subject to year-around drug testing (Elliott et al., 2021). Consequences for student athletes who fail these drug tests are set by the NCAA. When an individual tests positive for a banned substance, they lose their eligibility to compete (Elliott et al., 2018). The college or university may administer additional penalties.

The information the NCAA obtains from their substance abuse program and testing is published and disseminated for a variety of uses. NCAA research is important simply because, "substance use remains a leading cause of preventable death globally" (Bernstein, 2017, p. 1). It is vital to take any measure to ensure effective means of mitigating high-risk behaviors among NCAA student athletes and to prevent resulting adverse consequences, injury, and the possibility of death. Unlike the potential of injuries to athletes during practice and games, programs and education on substance abuse have the potential to prevent use by student athletes.

Testing for drug use by colleges and universities can vary depending on the administering body and their motivation for the substance abuse program. Some college and university athletic departments test in the same manner as the NCAA, for consideration for student athletes' well-being, while others use drug testing either as a form of deterrent to future use or in order to be more punitive, which results in suspension or expulsion (Elliott et al., 2018). No matter the motivation, coaches, trainers, college and university administrators, physicians, and others agree that substance use is an ongoing concern.

While drug testing aspires to be a deterrent from abuse, it is not the only intended outcome for this screening. Being drug free helps preserve the athletic abilities of student athletes. The research of Johnson et al. (2012) "confirm[s] athletic variables are powerfully linked to academic success" (p. 166), creating further benefits for the drug-free student athlete. While student athletes may tend not to use recreational drugs due to an adverse effect on performance, the use of ergogenic substances that improve performance may increase. No matter the drug of choice for a student athlete, the NCAA is determined to mitigate, if not eliminate, drug use among their student athlete cohort.

NCAA TESTING

The NCAA concern for the well-being of the student athlete clearly discourages alcohol and drug use in order to promote fair and safe competition for college athletes (Health & Safety, 2021). The problem is not isolated to NCAA student athletes; all collegiate athletes are expected to perform well enough in their studies to earn grades that support their eligibility to play their sport. During the season of a student athlete's sport, they often spend 20 or more hours in practice or actual play. They sustain bodily injury and fatigue and miss classes frequently (Gayles, 2009). These factors create a different experience than that of other students. The student athlete's sports participation can be impaired with drug use, and drug use can cause other types of sports-induced injury or exasperate existing physical conditions. These differences between student athletes and non-athletes will be further explored in the sections on culture and subcultures later in this chapter.

While participation in intercollegiate sports for student athletes has many positive, documented outcomes, research shows that student athletes engage in higher levels of risky behavior than their non-athletic peers (Graupensperger et al., 2018, p. 1). The NCAA oversight of the well-being and safety of student athletes takes risky behavior seriously, whether it occurs on or off the court. To achieve the best outcomes, the NCAA not only created their drug testing program, they developed clear policies and effective educational programs (NCAA Health and Safety, 2021).

Arguments exist in support of reform to the NCAA's drug testing policies. Because each college or university sets their own protocols for testing and for failed tests, a case could be made for a uniform policy with uniform frequency, counseling types, and duration and severity for penalties. The wide range of penalties enforced by NCAA institutions range from a one-year suspension to a 30-day suspension to missing 10% of the season or no suspension—all for a first positive drug screen (Elliott et al., 2018). Penalties differ, with one possible motivation being maintaining a student athlete's eligibility, to preserve a revenue-generating sport for the welfare of the college or university. Research by Elliott et al. (2018) indicated that "universities with more successful athletic programs had policies with more lenient penalties for suspension after each round of positive drug tests" (p. 36).

While the different consequences for failed drug testing indicate the need for uniformity in penalties across NCAA colleges and universities, a one-size-fits-all solution is also fraught with problems. First, there is lack of empirical investigation to determine the best approach to a universal drug testing policy.

The factors commonly debated about an appropriate methodology include fairness, frequency and rationale, and constraints for drug testing policies. Fairness would level the playing field since colleges and universities "seeking a competitive advantage may adopt weak testing policies to protect student-athlete eligibility" (Elliott et al., 2018, p. 26). The case for frequency allows testing to be used as a possible deterrent to student athletes' drug use. To further confound frequency is type, distinguishing between performance-enhancing drugs and recreational drugs. However, more frequent tests require greater expense and result in the possibility of more application of penalties. "Counseling sessions could be more expensive and out of reach for institutions with limited funding for such programs" (Elliott et al., 2018, p. 37). For rationale and constraints there are contradictions in existing research and literature. An empirical investigation on the topic of uniform drug testing programs that provides conclusive evidence does not yet exist. Because of this lack, the NCAA report continues to be a vital tool to scan for student athletes' substance abuse.

Along with the previous factors in testing is consideration for the development of overall penalties for infractions. Elliott et al. (2018) examined the possible sentences for positive drug tests, such as increased frequency of testing (after first positive test), counseling, suspension, dismissal (from team and/or college), along with the levels of penalties for first, second, or third infractions. The current penalties range from "zero-tolerance" policies to "second chance" policies and variations. The NCAA reported on those differences among member schools, and it is unclear why the variations exist. Without further research, it cannot be surmised whether policies are intentionally designed towards leniency or penalty.

Despite the longevity of the problem of substance abuse among student athletes and the current body of research, "future research is necessary to determine whether a uniform policy enforced by the NCAA would improve student-athlete wellness, curb the use of banned substances, and uphold the standards of fair play" (Elliott et al., 2018, p. 36). Without a uniform policy for NCAA member institutions, the existing autonomy of each college and university remains intact, with varying approaches to identification of substance abuse and resulting consequences.

CULTURE

Academic challenges, active and collaborative learning, student–faculty interaction, enriching educational experiences, and supportive campus environments are common among all students (Kuh, 2001), including the student athlete. The culture of a student athlete includes the overall campus environment and, depending on the perspective, the sports program or sports center can also be considered a culture with the various sport teams designated as subcultures. When athletic programs are considered as a culture, Gayle's (2009) research indicates "student-athletes experience lower levels of academic performance, graduate at lower rates, cluster in certain majors, and are socially segregated from the general student population" (p. 34).

The NCAA supports the integration of the student athlete into the general student population in order for them to benefit from all normative college experiences. The NCAA's drug testing program is intended to contribute to the campus environment in support of healthy choices and a positive environment for student athletes (NCAA Health and Safety, 2021). The learning experiences and personal growth of all types of student populations are rooted in good practices. Cultural norms that student-athletes encounter as part of the general culture include "these seven principles—interaction between faculty and students, cooperative learning among students, active learning, prompt feedback, time on task, communication of high expectations, and respect for diverse ways of learning" (NCAA Health and Safety, 2021). Because of these empirical findings, any form of athletic designation, either sports program or sports team, will be considered a *subculture* in this chapter. The general campus experience is considered the *culture*.

Substance abuse data indicates different results for student athletes compared to nonathletes use on campuses. It has been established that student athletes tend to represent a special population of students with unique challenges and needs that differ from their nonathletic peers" (Gayle, 2009). The duality of the student athlete creates two sets of unique challenges. They require support for two paths of success, academics and athletics. These two sets of demands can be difficult to balance. While colleges and universities provide support services and programs to ensure the success of their student bodies, Nite (2012) found that universities face certain challenges in supporting the overall development of their student athletes. Their role in athletic programs requires support and attention, especially in the area of substance abuse.

Rubin and Moses (2017) note, "Campus culture is often in conflict with the culture of the athletic department" (p. 325). The conflict is represented through the comparison of student athletes with non-student athletes in the area of alcohol and drug use, where student athletes (male) report more heavy drinking in the past year and more substance abuse in the form of banned performance-enhancing drugs, nutritional supplements, and smokeless tobacco (Yusko et al., 2008).

In any culture, there is a propensity to fit in or for "peer conformity." While some would posit that in the general student population, the student athlete enjoys an elite or high status standing, they are still exposed to prototypical behaviors. Student athletes may still be driven to conformity in various campus settings. These settings can also be considered subcultures of the culture and may include group membership with student housing, within their major, with Greek life, and most typically, with their sports team. The underlying motives for conforming are the same no matter the group: "(a) being socially accepted by group members and avoiding rejection, (b) establishing or maintaining self-concept as a member of the group, and (c) aligning with high status group members" (Graupensperger et al., 2018). Because of the significant influence subsets of students have on student athletes, the next section looks more closely at subculture's sway on the student-athlete in relation to substance abuse.

SUBCULTURE

The mission of higher education institutions does not include the creation of subcultures, specifically with regards to academics. From an academic standpoint, Gayles (2009) found that "student-athletes were as engaged in educational activities as compared to their nonathlete peers" (p. 39). However, studies about drug testing protocols and requirements showed differences between student athletes and nonathlete peers, as did the pattern of substance abuse between the two cohorts. Regarding testing protocols, there has been a long-standing concern about student athlete substance abuse (outlined in earlier sections). Regarding patterns of substance abuse, the motivation and actual participation in substance abuse varied for the two groups (student athlete versus nonathlete).

The nonathlete and the student athlete have distinct drug use encounters based on their different experiences. The student athlete has a unique college experience because they spend a portion of their time participating in sports activities. Student athletes miss out on many of the formative experiences that other students are exposed to. They may not be swayed by those general events like they are within their own athletic world. Existing research has shown that student athletes benefit as much from general college happenings as does the general student (Gayles, 2009). This has the potential to be used to improve the student athlete's practices with drug use while in the general population, not just within the realm of their team. There is more to be learned about the overall experience of the student athlete on the college campus.

It is known that the influence of the team culture on the student athlete provides greater susceptibility to substance abuse. Graupensperger et al. (2018) found that athletes altered their behavior to fit what they believed to be stereotypical behaviors of a group. That is not to say campus social norms do not contribute to substance abuse, but Zhou and Heim (2014) made a case that "sporting groups are suggested to be particularly peer-intensive and insular … due to the frequency of playing and training together" (p. 612). This means student athletes feel a strong pressure to engage in the same behaviors as teammates. This is important for the NCAA to leverage. While adverse effects originate from risky behavior, there is the potential application for beneficial behavior. This means the promotion of well-being and safety to student athletes can become exponential when the NCAA student athletes shun drug use and avail all of the benefits of their elite position.

SUMMARY

The NCAA student athlete can be considered an elite athlete with the untapped potential for lifelong success. In order to safeguard this valuable resource, the NCAA focuses on the three priorities of academics, well-being, and fairness. However, the NCAA has found continued challenges to the health and safety of the student athlete due to the prevalence of substance abuse. This enormous concern about drug use is not only because it can derail the student athlete during their college and athletic experience, but the negative impact can remain throughout their life and destroy future sports opportunities.

This chapter explored how the NCAA has reacted to substance abuse for more than 35 years. It is extremely sad and unfortunate that there is a continued need for diligence in drug testing of student athletes to detect and prevent substance abuse and deliver penalties. The NCAA's report provides an executive summary of their findings, detailing the percentage of student athletes' use of substances and breaking the overall results down by division, gender, and sport. Comparisons can be made to past reports to provide insight on progress or the need for more attentiveness to aspects of the problem. The most insightful portion of the report is the student athletes' personal substance abuse stories. The report documents the age when they first used drugs, how often they use drugs, the reason for drug use, the reason for not using drugs, their drug testing experiences and beliefs, and other personal motivations

(NCAA, 2012). This paper is recommended reading for more detailed comprehension about the NCAA's response to drug use among student athletes.

While it is true the campus culture and the subculture of athletic programs each contribute to student athletes' potential for risky behavior, it is also the place where education and prevention can occur. The impact of a campus culture and sport team subculture cannot be discounted; Graupensperger et al. (2018) discussed the importance of any set of behavioral standards for membership within a social category. The problem of substance abuse, whether the substances come from the general student body or other student athletes, relies on the influence of peers and the student athletes' susceptibility to engage (or not) in the drug activity (NCAA, 2012). The NCAA continues to support changing the social norms to change behaviors regarding drug use.

DISCUSSION QUESTIONS

1. What are the benefits and risks of creating a universal substance abuse policy for all colleges and universities?
2. Penalties for student athletes range from "zero tolerance" to "second chance" and variations in between. What do you consider the most appropriate approach?
3. How does the integration of the student athlete into the overall campus culture benefit them, and what are the risks?
4. Where do you think the greater susceptibility to encounter drug use occurs—with the general student population on campus or within the athletic department or team? Why?
5. Social norms on a campus or a sports team have a high level of influence over behaviors. How can the NCAA response leverage social norms to reduce risky substance abuse behaviors by student athletes?

REFERENCES

Bernstein, S. L., & D'Onofrio, G. (2017). Screening, treatment initiation, and referral for substance use disorders. *Addiction Science & Clinical Practice, 12*(1), 1–4.

Elliott, K., Kellison, T., & Cianfrone, B. (2018). NCAA drug testing policies and penalties: The role of team performance. *Journal of Intercollegiate Sport, 11,* 24–39.

Gayles, J. G. (2009). The student athlete experience. *New Directions for Institutional Research, 144,* 33–41.

Graupensperger, S. A., Benson, A. J., & Evans, M. B. (2018). Everyone else is doing it: The association between social identity and susceptibility to peer influence in NCAA athletes. *Journal of Sport and Exercise Psychology, 40*(3), 117–127.

Green, G. A., Uryasz, F. D., Petr, T. A., & Bray, C. D. (2001). NCAA study of substance use and abuse habits of college student-athletes. *Clinical Journal of Sport Medicine, 11*(1), 51–56.

Johnson, J. E., Wessel, R. D., & Pierce, D. A. (2012). The influence of selected variables on NCAA academic progress rate. *Journal of Issues in Intercollegiate Athletics, 5*, 149–171.

Kuh, G. D. (2001). Assessing what really matters to student learning: Inside the national survey of student engagement. *Change, 33*(3), 10–17.

National Collegiate Athletic Association (NCAA). (2012). *Substance use: National study of substance use trends among NCAA college student-athletes.* NCAAPublications.com

NCAA. (2021). What is the NCAA? https://www.ncaa.org/about/resources/media-center/ncaa-101/what-ncaa

NCAA Health and Safety. (2021). *Well-being.* https://www.ncaa.org/health-and-safety

Nite, C. (2012). Challenges for supporting student-athlete development: Perspectives from an NCAA Division II athletic department. *Journal of Issues in Intercollegiate Athletics, 5*, 1–14.

Rubin, L. M., & Moses, R. A. (2017). Athletic subculture within student-athlete academic centers. *Sociology of Sport Journal, 34*(4), 317–328.

Yusko, D. A., Buckman, J. F., White, H. R., & Pandina, R. J. (2008). Alcohol, tobacco, illicit drugs, and performance enhancers: A comparison of use by college student athletes and nonathletes. *Journal of American College Health, 57*(3), 281–290.

Zhou, J., & Heim, D. (2014). Sports and spirits: A systematic qualitative review of emergent theories for student-athlete drinking. *Alcohol and Alcoholism, 49*(6), 604–617.

The Treatment Process When Working With Athletes Who Misuse Drugs

INTRODUCTION

Drug use in America is a topic that instantly generates discussion, but when athletes are included in the discussion, solutions are suggested that do not focus on the wellness or well-being of the athlete. The focus is generally on the sport played by the athlete and what is to happen to the sport or what is to happen to the trophies or medals that the athlete has accumulated. While the majority of the content of this book focuses on the sport, this chapter provides a cursory view from the lens of the treatment process. Due to the nature of the world of sports, it is reasonable to state that every athlete at some point in their athletic career has been exposed to either abuse or misuse of drugs within their team. Although many athletes do not abuse drugs, many do, and the concern is that many of them do not receive the type of assistance needed to overcome their struggle. They may not receive assistance because they do not identify as experiencing a drug problem or because coaches and trainers may play a role in the abuse either intentionally or unintentionally. At other times the problem may be known but not addressed due to stigma. Athletes' quest to "be the best" is one of the major underlying causes for their drug abuse (Reardon & Creado, 2014). Even though doping is considered a public health issue, according to the CDC, many athletes do not receive treatment. This is an area of contradictions because millions of dollars are spent on training equipment and technological sensor devices to monitor and measure performance, yet little attention is given to the mental health and substance use disorders of athletes. Surveys seem to document the use across every sport, varying with gender, race, and specific drugs.

NCAA conducts a survey every 4 years on substance use habits of division athletes. The 2018 survey suggests decreases ("down slightly from previous years") in the use of alcohol. Tobacco use decreased slightly. Marijuana use was higher among student athletes living in states where recreational and medicinal use is legal, and all sport marijuana use was higher among male athletes. Division III student athletes also reported higher usage of marijuana. Amphetamine use has decreased since 2013. Lacrosse athletes reported the highest rate of cocaine use, which is similar to the 2013 survey report. Meanwhile, use of non-prescribed narcotic pain medication decreased.

Figure 8.1 provides data for a 2014 survey. Yet during the pandemic crisis for the period of 2020–2021, there was an increase in addiction deaths, emergency visits, and overdoses related to alcohol and other drugs (Shatterproof, 2021).

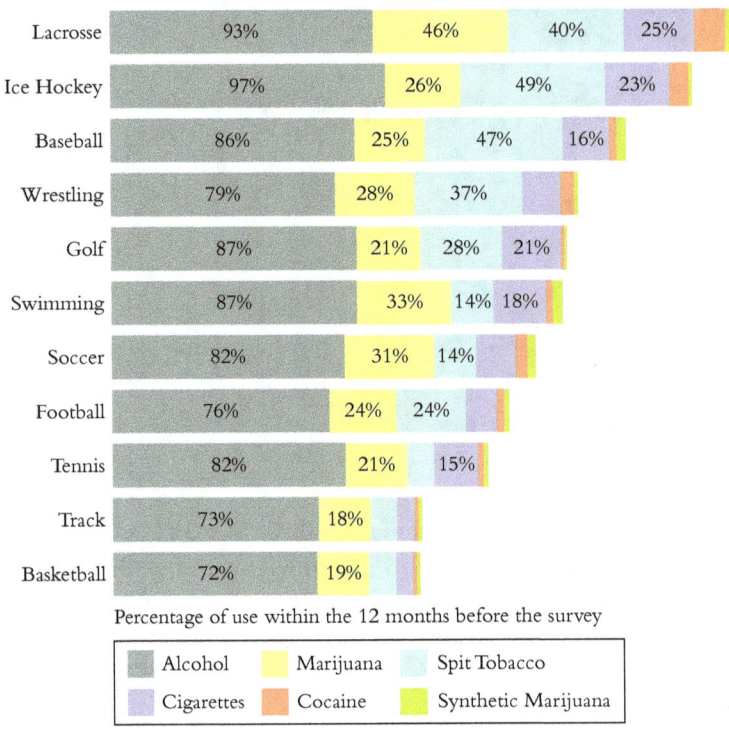

FIGURE 8.1 *College Athlete Substance Use, by Men's Sport*

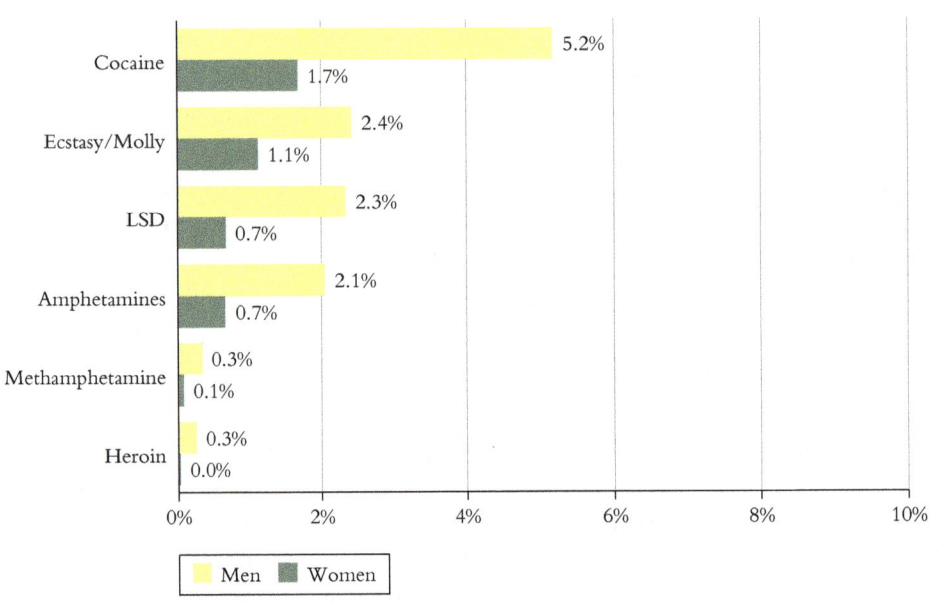

FIGURE 8.2 *Illicit Drug Use in the Last Year*

82 | Mental Health and Substance Use Disorders Among Athletes

As can be seen with the figures, the abuse of drugs is in every sport and not limited to illegal drugs. Prescription drugs and dietary supplements are also abused in sport. Many of the athletes abuse substances because they want to win and drugs provide them with the edge needed to perform well. Other reasons that they may abuse substances are to relieve pain from injury, to quickly recover from an injury, or due to stressors such as family issues, poor academic performance which may cause ineligibility, and extreme competition in the sport. Each rationale for the use of drugs points to the major rationale of the desire to perform well, with winning as the final outcome. Doping, as it is referred to in the sport world, is commonplace, and athletes will continue to become creative with the use of prohibited drugs, keeping in step with technological drug detection devices (Reardon & Creado, 2014). However, treatment is seldom mentioned or offered by the sport's team. NCAA mandates drug testing—but not treatment—if an athlete screens positive. Doping has always existed in sports and will continue to exist, but the anticipation is that treatment should be given equal attention within athletic departments.

ADDICTION TREATMENT FOR STUDENT ATHLETES

Although there are prevention campaigns on most collegiate campuses, many student athletes do not notice campus activities due to their rigorous training schedules. Also, some student athletes may feel that there is no need to pay attention to prevention because doping is considered "normal" within the ranks of the sport. Medical doctors, coaches, and trainers provide PEDs to care for injuries and obtain a quick recovery so that the athlete can reenter the game without delay. The game is the priority, but what about the athlete? While the coaches and trainers are considering the next athlete to replace the injured athlete, the injured athlete is considering whether the injury will end their career, end the collegiate experience, let down the team, along with feeling shame for allowing the injury to occur. These pressures can cause the athlete to become depressed and can move some athletes into using more PEDs to expedite the recovery process and relieve the pain (both physical and psychological). This mindset and action can lead to abuse of drugs.

Addressing the Drug Abuse Among Athletes

All counselors are not equipped to provide substance use disorder counseling. This implies that counselors should not practice beyond the scope of their specialty. Substance use and addiction counselors are licensed to provide counseling in this area of specialty. Thus, athletic departments should ensure that a licensed counselor works with athletes who are experiencing drug-related problems. Although there will be differences in how these counselors approach the issues, it is clear that the licensed counselor enters with a set of foundational competencies that focus on guidelines that are ethical and respectful of each client. A major shortcoming of past substance abuse treatments has been in the unidimensional thinking that substance abuse or addiction only occurs in poverty-stricken areas and among truly disadvantaged populations. Thus, counselors were armed with moral judgement and confrontational approaches to counseling (Lewis, Dana, & Blevins, 2002). However, more recent best practices suggest multidimensional approaches to the treatment process of substance abuse and addiction, beginning with understanding the 12 core functions in the treatment process:

Screening—The first step is to determine if the client is appropriate and eligible for services. The counselor decides if the client has abused a drug and identifies specific behaviors that would provide evidence that abuse has/is occurring, which is cause for dysfunction. The appropriateness of the client's program is based on the counselor's judgment (e.g., inpatient, outpatient, day care, detoxification). The counselor is responsible for not only making judgment calls based on their practice skills, but also providing suggestions or alternatives that are in the best interests of the client.

Intake—An administrative procedure where the client completes paperwork. Release of information and consent for treatment are essential forms that should be completed during the intake. Insurance information and the assignment of a counselor occurs.

Orientation—Client's rights are discussed along with the policies and procedures for treatment, which include discharge and termination policies. Also, information is provided regarding what to do in case of an emergency.

Assessment—The counselor provides information regarding the client's problem (identification of the problem), the client's strengths and weaknesses, and the considerations of the focus (goals and objectives) for the treatment plan. The assessment should be inclusive of major biopsychosocial areas: physical health, psychological functioning, social functioning, and legal aspects.

Treatment plan—The counselor and the client should work together to create a prioritized list of problem areas and to develop long-term and short-term goals and objectives. Resources should also be identified, including roles and responsibilities (who will provide services), frequency, and time frames for accomplishing specific objectives.

Counseling—The counselor must use special skills in group, individual, and family counseling to assist the client with resolving their problem. Thus, the counselor will have to understand and be able to apply diverse counseling approaches (e.g., reality therapy, motivational interviewing, or client-centered). The counselor must remember that theory guides practice and must be able to provide logical rationale for the treatment approach.

Case management—Coordinates and contacts other agencies and people who can assist with plans of action to meet the client's goals.

Crisis intervention—A critical event that occurs during the counseling process that may directly involve the drug use (e.g., relapse) or be indirectly related (e.g., death of family member). The critical event will be cause for immediate intervention. The crisis can be used by the counselor to move the treatment process forward.

Client education—Clients are provided information about drugs and their impact on lives, as well as other resources that may prove beneficial to the client.

Referral—If the counselor cannot meet the client's needs, other community resources should be sought. During the referral process, the counselor must adhere to confidentiality, ensuring that the client's privacy is safeguarded.

Report and recordkeeping—Maintaining the clinical notes, assessment reports, and discharge and termination information. All written information about the client must be maintained and safeguarded.

Consultation with other professionals—Meeting (face-to-face or virtual) to discuss the treatment and other decisions about the client. Typically, treatment teams will meet monthly (more times as needed depending on the client) to discuss the client's progression and future prognosis. Meeting with a supervisor about a case is also considered consultation. These meetings may occur weekly, depending on the client and the level of practice of the counselor.

In order to obtain a license in addiction counseling, counselors must demonstrate proficiency in these 12 core areas of practice. These 12 core functions were developed in 1980 by a group of representatives from different states to address the competency skill levels of substance abuse counselors (Parisi, n.d.). Many professional programs, such as graduate social work (MSW) programs, do not include specific substance abuse education in their academic curricula, which can lead to misdiagnosis and lack of competency for working with this population (Johnson, 2012). Yet social workers are primary counselors and considered frontline counselors in times of crises (including substance abuse crisis situations). Therefore, it is essential that the counselor does not practice outside their scope of practice. The scope of practice includes the services or the intervention approaches that a counselor is authorized to accomplish with clients, based on their license to practice. The license to practice signifies that the counselor is competent (educated and trained) in specific specialty areas. It is essential to realize the importance of taking appropriate steps if a client's needs are outside the scope of practice so that no harm is caused to the client. This can be determined by the counselor at the point of screening, intake, and assessment. For example, if a social worker receives a call that an athlete needs counseling due to admission of an active illegal drug problem, and the social worker has no training in addiction counseling, it would be wise to refer the athlete to a counselor with addictions as a scope of practice. Because social workers do not possess skill sets in all levels of practice, referrals or consultations are useful.

Initial client referrals (no contact with the client—phone or written report referrals) are not as complicated as referrals after a few sessions with a client. If discovery is made that a referral is appropriate because of information that is outside the scope of the counselor, it is important to discuss this with the client and supervisor and then seek resources (counselors who specialize) and make the referral. This is suggested because the termination process is equally important as the initial session with the client in the therapeutic process (DeAngelis, 2018). The termination process allows the client to reflect with the counselor on future goals and objectives, but also sends the message to the client that the termination occurs not because of the client but because the client progressed to a point in therapy where another counselor can become more helpful to the client. In this manner, the client does not feel blame for the referral, and the counselor should not feel shame. Some well-intended counselors may be asked to perform duties outside their skill set. If in doubt, seek advice (Rimmer, 2021). Although states laws may differ regarding licensure, it is important to understand that counseling outside the scope of practice can be subject to disciplinary hearing and result in license suspension or revocation by the granting state board.

In an effort to assist practitioners to expand their scope of practice, SAMHSA has provided funds to increase the education and skills of medical doctors, nurses, and health care providers, specifically in the areas of substance use disorders and including prescription drugs. For example, Project Result was designed by the George Washington University School of Medicine and Health Sciences. The project started in August 2021 and will end September 1, 2023. The overall aim is to "provide a practical, succinct overview of addiction as a brain disease, screening, brief intervention and treatment and referral for care. Throughout the training we provide links to additional resources should you want to dive deeper into any of these topics" (GWU, 2021, para. 2).

Drug addiction treatment can include a wide scope of practice. NIDA (2020) suggests that treatment can range from medications (e.g., methadone and naltrexone) to behavioral therapies (e.g., CBT or contingency management) or a combination of treatment approaches. The specific type of treatment approach will depend on the individual client, frequency of use, and type of drug.

PREVENTION, POLICIES, AND POLITICS

Prevention begins with the need to provide relevant and accurate information to individuals, groups, and community. Substance abuse/misuse and disorders are public health concerns. Appropriate prevention can cause shifts in public health concerns. SAMHSA (2016) noted that there has been a shift in the leading causes of death based on prevention effort reports. Citing the 20th century's leading causes of death from infectious diseases (tuberculosis) and noncommunicable diseases (diabetes and cancer) shifting to health issues such as substance use, violence, and mental health in the 21st century as leading causes of death.

Policies that focus on alcohol misuse have proven effective and demonstrated a reduction in the misuse (SAMHSA, 2016). However, evidence is mixed and inconclusive on the misuse of illegal and prescription drugs. Griffin and Botvin (2010) note that risk and protective factors are contributing features of the initiation, maintenance, and continuation of alcohol and drug misuse/abuse. In the sports world, risk and protective factors may appear to be the same, which presents a rather confusing picture for the athlete. For example, a risk factor may be the athlete who enters college away from home for the first time and is a witness to teammates using drugs (alcohol and marijuana) so to fit in he will also join. The protective factor should theoretically be the coach and training staff; however, they exacerbate the situation with the inclusion of PEDs to enhance the athlete's performance or to hasten quick injury recovery. Totally confused, the athlete cannot discuss this situation with parents or family members and all of the "friends" are teammates. NCAA policies provide a list of prohibited drugs, but the athlete has been thrown into a pit of confusion with the only way out silent conformity. All this places the athlete at greater risk of becoming depressed or isolated and eventually addicted.

When money is involved, the issue becomes political and one has to break from the excitement of the sport and wonder if the monetary gains are worth the well-being and careers and lives of collegiate athletes. Who are the winners when it comes to policy and decision-making about PEDs? We know that coaches are the winners with increased salaries if their teams win, but there is seldom mention of the pharmaceutical companies who manufacture and distribute the drugs. They are likely the biggest winners of the group. These companies market many dietary supplements to athletes, suggesting that the supplements have an ergogenic impact on their bodies (Ambrose, 2004). Although many of the supplements are banned or placed on prohibited lists, the pharmaceutical companies continue to participate in the doping of athletes with their sales pitches and advertisements. If there was truly an urge to discontinue, or at least to reduce the doping among collegiate athletes, a beginning would be pharmaceutical companies limiting their access to coaches, training staff, and athletes as buyers of their supplements. This is unlikely to occur because of the large monetary loss that would be suffered by these companies. The issue continues to be that the individuals with the most power (money) to stop the distribution and purchase of PEDs would be the companies that will not risk suffering a financial loss, regardless of the loss of collegiate student athletes' careers and lives.

SIGNS AND SYMPTOMS

The Mayo Clinic (2021) provides a detailed synopsis of the signs and symptoms for prescription drug misuse and abuse. Collegiate athletes sometimes unintentionally abuse prescription drugs in their quest to recover faster. They do not realize the consequences of the misuse or abuse of the prescribed medication(s).

The following are the most commonly abused prescription drugs:

- **Opioids**, medications containing oxycodone—such as Oxycontin and Percocet—and those containing hydrocodone—such as Norco. Used to treat pain.
- **Anti-anxiety medications and sedatives**, such as alprazolam (Xanax) and diazepam (Valium).
- **Hypnotics**, such as zolpidem (Ambien). Used to treat anxiety and sleep disorders.
- **Stimulants**, such as methylphenidate (Ritalin, Concerta, others), dextroamphetamine/amphetamine (Adderall XR, Mydayis), and dextroamphetamine (Dexedrine). Used to treat attention-deficit/hyperactivity disorder (ADHD) and certain sleep disorders.

Source: Prescription drug abuse—Symptoms and causes—Mayo Clinic, https://www.mayoclinic.org/diseases-conditions/prescription-drug-abuse/symptoms-causes/syc-20376813

TABLE 8.1 Signs and Symptoms of Prescription Drug Abuse

Opioids	Anti-anxiety Medications and Sedatives	Stimulants
- Constipation - Nausea - Feeling high (euphoria) - Slowed breathing rate - Drowsiness - Confusion - Poor coordination - Increased dose required for pain relief - Worsening or increased sensitivity to pain with higher doses (hyperalgesia)	- Drowsiness - Confusion - Unsteady walking - Slurred speech - Poor concentration - Dizziness - Problems with memory - Slowed breathing	- Increased alertness - Feeling high - Irregular heartbeat - High blood pressure - High body temperature - Reduced appetite - Insomnia - Agitation - Anxiety - Paranoia

Other signs include:

- Stealing, forging or selling prescriptions
- Taking higher doses than prescribed
- Excessive mood swings or hostility
- Increase or decrease in sleep
- Poor decision-making
- Appearing to be high, unusually energetic or revved up, or sedated
- Requesting early refills or continually "losing" prescriptions, so more prescriptions must be written
- Seeking prescriptions from more than one doctor

Source: Prescription drug abuse—Symptoms and causes, Mayo Clinic, https://www.mayoclinic.org/diseases-conditions/prescription-drug-abuse/symptoms-causes/syc-20376813

INTERVENTION STRATEGIES

One size does not fit all, and therefore, intervention strategies must be considered based on client needs. Some effective (evidence-based) strategies are delineated, but consideration should be given to individual needs and focus. Brief intervention strategies have been used by practitioners with at-risk clients and those with less severe abuse behaviors. These strategies are structured, time limited, and directed toward a specific goal (Center for Substance Abuse Treatment, 1999). Some examples of brief intervention techniques are abstaining, self-help support groups (12-step programs), and individual brief counseling.

Lal and Singh (2018) provide a list of tools that can be used for assessment purposes. Many of these instruments are utilized in clinical practice as screening and or assessment tools. The actual survey or questionnaires can be obtained online without charge. These instruments have been empirically proven to be effective tools that are acceptable for use with clients. They can strengthen the continuum of care features that are delineated by ASAM guidelines.

American Society of Addiction Medicine (ASAM) is a physician lead organization of about 3,000 physicians and associate members with the focus on "full spectrum of addiction care," which includes continuity of care guidelines. The spectrum of care is based on prevention, treatment, remission, and recovery, according to the 2018–2021 strategic plan (ASAM, 2021). The ASAM criteria are the most widely used guidelines for providing assessments, planning, placement, and discharge for those clients who have addictive disorders (Mee-Lee, 2015).

The ASAM commitment is to fund and engage in research and training that will focus on treating addictions, improving health and saving lives. ASAM dating back in the 1980s developed one national set of criteria as a result of a collaborative process with doctors, social workers, and psychologists discussing and providing feedback from treatment. Community coalitions came together to support the ASAM criteria. The goal is to unify the addiction field under a single set of criteria. Used in over 30 states and in the department of defense in other countries (e.g., Norway) (Mee-Lee, 2015), the ASAM provides a multidimensional vision, looking at the whole person and describing a continuation of care.

The criteria do not provide a checklist, but severity and levels of functioning are delineated. It is essential to provide clients with complete care. Thus, the focus should not only include physical and mental health care, but substance abuse care as well.

Lo et al. (2020) suggest that substance abuse is a chronic relapsing disease requiring multilevel interventions. Although their suggestion to consider many different aspects such as "psychological, personality, cognitive, socioeconomic, familial and cultural differences of various social groups," their recommendation is based on unidimensional methodology (quantitative design). If a multilevel perspective is to be introduced, every aspect of the paradigm should reflect multilevel approaches. It is significant and relevant to obtain information based on the client's perspectives. Often missing from the research on substance use and misuse is the client's reasoning. Thus, the inclusion of more qualitative research designs would prove useful, especially when working with athletes.

Brief interventions are offered as a beginning exploration of the intervention feature of counseling. These interventions are typically evidence-based (have been scientifically proven effective) and are widely used by addiction counselors. They include crisis intervention, individual therapy, group therapy, brief therapy, multicultural approaches, relapse models, and harm reduction model. One of the most popular is cognitive behavior therapy (CBT), a short term (12- to 24-week) therapeutic intervention that has been deemed effective for treating substance misuse and disorders in athletes (SAMHSA, 2016). CBT is founded on the premise that behavior and dysfunctional thinking are reasons for substance misuse/abuse. Thus, the modification of behavior and thinking is needed. The focus of counseling is on the substance misuse/abuse while weighing the pros and cons of continuing the use.

Motivational interviewing (MI) is another typical approach used by addiction counselors. MI is similar to Carl Rogers's client-centered approach, where the client's ambivalence to change is a focus in counseling. However, unlike Rogers's approach where the client guides the process, in MI the counselor is more directive in assisting the clients to reach their goal(s) (SAMHSA, 2016). MI has been suggested as one of the best intervention approaches for treating athletes because athletes may typically present in the precontemplation stage of change (Reardon & Creado, 2014). They suggest the following for elements of MI should be significant considerations when working with athletes:

Clinician empathy, which is comprised of reflective listening and language style, is a significant factor in maintaining a positive therapeutic alliance (Lord et al., 2015).

Developing discrepancies between the impact of continued use of substances and the goal after the sport. During this process, the provider helps athletes to clarify conflict among their values, motives, interests, and behaviors.

Rolling with resistance rather than arguing with the athlete because the argument can prolong resistance to change. The counselor can "agree to disagree" on certain points with some athletes, or the counselor may "wonder about" certain alternative actions, but they do not impose or insist upon their perspective.

Encourage self-efficacy. Athletes may need to change their thinking from "winning is everything" or willingness to do anything to win (misusing PEDs). If an athlete is dependent on a drug (addicted), numerous strategies such as pharmacologic interventions (naltrexone, disulfiram, buprenorphine) may be needed. Counselors should assess for comorbid mental illness, since co-occurrence of physical dependence and mental illness is commonplace. Cognitive behavioral therapy, 12-step programs, and network therapy are also approaches that may be helpful for athletes who are abusing drugs, although studies are preliminary (Reardon & Creado, 2014).

Although there are numerous evidence-based intervention strategies, however, a major concern is that interventions and programs are not capturing athletes into counseling and programs. This is largely due to the factors such as stigma, time frame for program attendance, and program staff not reaching out to the athletic department as collaborators. In order to provide successful intervention (success as defined by recruitment and retainment) of athletes who misuse drugs, it is essential to collaborate with the coaches and training staff, especially during the initial phrase of the program development process. However, "reaching out" to coaches and training staff may produce additional dilemmas for the counselor and the athletes, especially in the area of confidentiality and privacy.

FEDERAL LAWS

HIPAA

The Health Insurance Portability and Accountability Act [1996] was established based on the need to keep and maintain health information as a private. The overall goal is to protect clients' health information. This is inclusive of electronic medical records (Edemekong et al., 2021). In addition to protecting the client's health information, the HIPAA Privacy Rule allows client access to the file. Clients can obtain copies of their records by requesting in writing a copy of their personal file. The agency or private provider must respond (provide the file) within 30 days. Writing an incorrect name or address, phone number, or email, or discussing information publicly can be deemed HIPAA violations with harsh consequences.

Title 42 CFR Part 2

Title 42 of the Code of Federal Regulations Part 2 (42 CFR Part 2) controls the release of patient information about treatment for substance use disorders. The purpose of the law is to decrease the release of information about individuals who are in recovery so that these individuals will not suffer from discrimination and more individuals can seek and receive treatment for the disorder (Brooks, 2000). Any program or private practitioner that provides assessment, treatment, counseling, or referrals related to substance abuse disorders or misuse must comply with federal restrictions contained in this law. These federal laws are to protect the client, but the client can sign release of information forms to allow information to be released to specific entities. The information can only be released to the entity or entities listed on the signed release form. The consent form for the release of information must contain the following:

- the name or general description of the program(s) making the disclosure;
- the name or title of the individual or organization that will receive the disclosure;

- the name of the client who is the subject of the disclosure;
- the purpose or need for the disclosure;
- how much and what kind of information will be disclosed;
- a statement that the client may revoke (take back) the consent at any time, except to the extent that the program has already acted on it;
- the date, event, or condition upon which the consent will expire if not previously revoked;
- the signature of the client (and, in some states, that of the parent); and
- the date on which the consent is signed (Brooks, 2000).

A client has a right to revoke their consent at any time. Although verbal request to revoke is acceptable, it is best to obtain a written statement of the request so that a copy can be maintained in the client's file.

These two federal laws are cause for notice by counselor especially those working with athletes. Athletes have a special bond with their coach and training staff. The coach feels the need to know all information about their players, especially if may impact the athlete's playing. However, the federal laws are very strict about issues related to medical information and information about substance abuse disorders. Not providing information to coaches may result in the athlete's removal from the team, but revealing information may result in the counselor having their license revoked. It is important for counselors to review the HIPAA guidelines and 42 CFR Part A if they work with substance misusing/abusing athletes.

SUMMARY

Although many prevention and intervention strategies have demonstrated effectiveness, the concern is that these programs are not used by populations most in need. For example, athletes are not using these programs. Many counselors (specifically social workers) are not using effective intervention strategies because they are either outside of their scope of practice, or the athletes do not participate in the program or in counseling. Further, many of these programs are designed by researchers who have limited knowledge about the client target population (athletes). Therefore, the cultural factor is lost in the process, and thus, the program either does not meet the goals and objectives defined or program attrition causes a major limitation in the research study process. Increasing the number of social work researchers who are knowledgeable about sports and athletes will yield meaningful research while providing significant and relevant treatment for this underserved treatment population.

DISCUSSION QUESTIONS

1. In a group, identify some substance programs that are considered effective and then discuss whether athletes attend the programs. Discuss why or why not.
2. Coaches and trainers have been identified both as a risk factor and as a protective factor. Explain this by providing examples.

3. Go to the internet and identify one "popular" alcohol and illegal drug screening instrument. After reviewing the instrument, explain what modifications would be needed to administer it to an athlete.
4. In a group, identify an athlete who has been affected by substance misuse. Discuss the consequences and how the policy impacted the consequences.
5. Many athletes do not receive treatment for substance misuse/abuse. List three reasons for the lack of treatment. Then explain how these reasons for lack of treatment can be overcome for future athletes.

REFERENCES

Ambrose, P. J. (2004). Drug use in sports: A veritable arena for pharmacists. *Journal of the American Pharmacists Association, 44*(4), 501–514; quiz 514–516. doi: 10.1331/1544345041475698. PMID: 15372871

ASAM. (2021). *Strategic plan 2018–2021.* asam.org

Brooks, M. (2000). *Substance abuse treatment for persons with child abuse and neglect issues* (Appendix B: Protecting clients' privacy). Center for Substance Abuse Treatment. Substance Abuse and Mental Health Services Administration (US). https://www.ncbi.nlm.nih.gov/books/NBK64900/

Center for Substance Abuse Treatment. (1999). Brief interventions in substance abuse treatment. In Treatment Improvement Protocol (TIP) Series, No. 34. Substance Abuse and Mental Health Services Administration (US). https://www.ncbi.nlm.nih.gov/books/NBK64942/

DeAngelis, T. (2018). What should you do if a case is outside your skill set? *American Psychological Association, 49*(5). https://www.apa.org/monitor/2018/05/ce-corner

Edemekong, P. F., Annamaraju, P., & Haydel, M. J. (2021). *Health Insurance Portability and Accountability Act.* [Updated February 3, 2021]. StatPearls Publishing. https://www.ncbi.nlm.nih.gov/books/NBK500019/

George Washington University. (2021). Project RESULT: Rethinking Substance Use Disorder Practitioner Learning and Teaching. https://cme.smhs.gwu.edu/content/project-result#group-tabs-node-course-default1?utm_source=google&utm_medium=ppc&utm_campaign=LMO-SMHS-TRAINING-FY22

Griffin, K. W., & Botvin, G. J. (2010). Evidence-based interventions for preventing substance use disorders in adolescents. *Child and Adolescent Psychiatric Clinics of North America, 19*(3), 505–526. https://doi.org/10.1016/j.chc.2010.03.005

Johnson, A. (2012). *Substance abuse education in master's of social work programs: A content analysis.* Sophia, St. Catherine University repository website: https://sophia.stkate.edu/msw_papers/126

Lal, R., & Singh, S. (2018). Assessment tools for screening and clinical evaluation of psychosocial aspects in addictive disorders. *Indian Journal of Psychiatry, 60*(Suppl 4), S444–S450. https://doi.org/10.4103/psychiatry.IndianJPsychiatry_12_18; https://www.ncbi.nlm.nih.gov/pmc/articles/PMC5844153/

Lewis, J. A., Dana, R. Q., & Blevins, G. A. (2002). *Substance abuse counseling* (3rd ed.). Brooks/Cole.

Lo, T. W., Yeung, J., & Tam, C. (2020). Substance abuse and public health: A multilevel perspective and multiple responses. *International Journal of Environmental Research and Public Health, 17*(7), 2610. https://doi.org/10.3390/ijerph17072610

Lord, S. P., Sheng, E., Imel, Z. E., Baer, J., & Atkins, D. C. (2015). More than reflections: empathy in motivational interviewing includes language style synchrony between therapist and client. *Behavior Therapy, 46*(3), 296–303. https://doi.org/10.1016/j.beth.2014.11.002

Mayo Clinic. (2021). Prescription drug abuse. https://www.mayoclinic.org/diseases-conditions/prescription-drug-abuse/symptoms-causes/syc-20376813

Mee-Lee, D. (2015). Understanding the new ASAM criteria. NAADAC. naadac.org

NCAA. (2018). *NCAA student-athlete substance use study: Executive summary, June 2018.* https://ncaaorg.s3.amazonaws.com/research/substance/2017RES_SubstanceUseExecutiveSummary.pdf

NIDA. (2020, September 18). Frequently asked questions: What is drug addiction treatment? https://nida.nih.gov/sites/default/files/podat-3rdEd-508.pdf

Parisi, D. (n.d.). *The twelve core functions of the substance use counselor.* https://www.mass.gov/doc/core-functions/download

Reardon, C. L., & Creado, S. (2014). Drug abuse in athletes. *Substance Abuse and Rehabilitation, 5,* 95–105. https://doi.org/10.2147/SAR.S53784; https://www.ncbi.nlm.nih.gov/pmc/articles/PMC4140700/

Rimmer, A. (2021). What should I do if I'm asked to work outside of my practice? *BMJ, 372*(586). https://doi.org/10.1136/bmj.n586; https://www.bmj.com/content/372/bmj.n586

Shatterproof. (2021). Addiction is a public health crisis. shatterproof.org

Substance Abuse and Mental Health Services Administration (SAMHSA). (2016). Prevention programs and polices. In Office of the Surgeon General (US), *Facing addiction in America: The Surgeon General's report on alcohol, drugs, and health* [Internet]. U.S. Department of Health and Human Services. https://www.ncbi.nlm.nih.gov/books/NBK424850/

IMAGE CREDITS

Fig. 8.1: Source: Adapted from https://projectknow.com/discover/college-athletes-and-substance-use/.

Fig. 8.2: Source: https://ncaaorg.s3.amazonaws.com/research/substance/2017RES_SubstanceUseExecutiveSummary.pdf.

Injuries as the Ultimate Gateway Drug

INTRODUCTION

Performing as an athlete is often accompanied by high levels of pressure and stress. Athletes typically strive for high levels of perfection due to the expectations for high performance standards (Hauck et al., 2020, p. 115). Due to high levels of pressure, and other elements such as injuries, it is common for athletes to develop co-occurring disorders. Various mental health symptoms and disorders have been noted among the athletic population, including depression, anxiety, distress, and substance misuse (Gouttebarge et al., 2019, p. 700). The prevalence of mental health disorders has been found to be approximately the same as what is noted in the general population, making the challenge important to address (Gouttebarge et al., 2019, p. 700). In addition, exercise addiction and food addiction have been identified as common mental health disorders impacting the athletic population in recent years (Levit et al., 2018, p. 1). Each of these disorders has the potential to occur simultaneously, creating co-occurring disorders.

Injuries have been described as one of the highest risk factors for psychological ailments among athletes (Souter et al., 2018, p. 2). To effectively combat these challenges, athletes often benefit from counseling services. However, barriers exist to providing athletes with counseling, including the presence of masculinity, personal attitudes toward mental health care, the ability to receive care, and the attitudes of parents, teammates, coaches, and trainers (Moreland et al., 2018, p. 65). Alternatively, these same factors can increase the likelihood of the athlete receiving mental health care (Moreland et al., 2018, p. 65). This chapter aims to explore co-occurring disorders among athletes, including anxiety and depression disorders, eating and exercise disorders, and substance use disorder, and the role of injuries in developing co-occurring disorders. In addition, it will describe how counseling can be a vital tool to athletes and their overall well-being.

CO-OCCURRING DISORDERS AMONG ATHLETES

Athletes are prone to experiencing a variety of co-occurring disorders. One study noted that the prevalence of co-occurring mental health disorders is the same in athletes and the general population (Gouttebarge et al., 2019, p. 700). These individuals often experience a variety of mental distress symptoms, including the onset of depression, anxiety, and substance use disorder (Gouttebarge et al., 2019, p. 700). High levels of pressure, stress, and the desire for perfectionism can exacerbate the challenges faced by athletes and result in eating and exercise disorders (Hauck et al., 2020, pp. 114–115). Often, the risk of onset of these conditions is heightened when transitioning out of the sport (Gouttebarge et al., 2019, p. 700). Also, the onset of injuries can significantly impact the athlete, resulting in depression (Souter et al., 2018). Injuries can require rehabilitation services and spur the onset of "self-treatment" through substance misuse (Gil et al., 2016, p. 1; Gouttebarge et al., 2019, p. 705). The following sections will examine in-depth co-occurring disorders such as anxiety and depression, eating disorders and exercise disorders, and the onset of substance use disorder, which can co-occur with multiple mental health disorders.

Anxiety and Depression

Mental health issues vary from individual to individual. The onset of anxiety and depression are among the most common reported mental health issues (Souter et al., 2018, p. 2). Athletes participating and competing in individual sports have been found to be more likely to experience the onset of anxiety and depression than their peers participating in team sports (Levit et al., 2018, p. 801). These disorders may include a variety of conditions, including generalized anxiety disorder (GAD), depressive disorder, obsessive-compulsive disorder (OCD), and social anxiety disorder (SAD), among other depression or phobia-based conditions (Souter et al., 2018, p. 2). Additionally, athletes with anxiety and depression disorders and symptoms also often experience sleep disturbances and various types of mental distress (Gouttebarge et al., 2019, p. 701). Anxiety and depression disorders have been noted to co-occur with eating disorders and addiction disorders, including substance use disorder (Levit et al., 2018, p. 803). Female athletes with anxiety and depression symptoms are noted to have a prevalence of 1% for bulimia nervosa (BN) and 4% for anorexia nervosa (AN), which create a co-occurring challenge requiring intervention (Gouttebarge et al., 2019, p. 701). Moreover, athletes suffering from anxiety and depression issues often develop alcohol misuse to cope with the challenging symptoms (Gouttebarge et al., 2019, p. 701). The presence of anxiety and depressive disorders can, therefore, have major impacts on the well-being and functioning of athletes and increase the risk of developing co-occurring challenges.

Eating and Exercise Disorders

Perfectionism is commonly noted among athletes. In these cases, the individual strives for "flawlessness and setting exceedingly high standards of performance," while often also being highly critical of their performance (Hauck et al., 2020, p. 115). The presence of perfectionism has been associated with the development of negative behaviors, including problematic exercising, and eating disorders (Hauck et al., 2020, p. 114). This includes the development of food addictions, binge eating disorder (BED), bulimia nervosa (BN), and anorexia nervosa (AN) (Hauck et al., 2020, p. 114). Eating disorders can include the restriction of eating and abnormal eating behaviors and is often attributed to goals pertaining to establishing and maintaining a certain weight required for the sport (Souter et al., 2018, p. 4). However, in cases of binge eating, it is common for individuals to have food addictions in which they overconsume and then attempt to compensate through excessive exercise (Hauck et al., 2020, p. 115). Regardless of the type of eating disorder, each is problematic and requires effective treatment modalities.

The presence of eating disorders in athletes is often accompanied by exercise addiction and the desire to achieve a particular body shape (Levit et al., 2018, p. 801). Additionally, the onset of eating disorders among athletes is also identified as a risk factor in developing other mental health disorders, creating an additional co-occurring condition (Souter et al., 2018, p. 3). Females often demonstrate a higher risk for exercise and eating disorders than their male athletic counterparts (Levit et al., 2018, p. 802). However, male elite athletes are more prone to developing eating disorders than males in the general population (Souter et al., 2018, p. 4). Therefore, eating and exercising disorders are important psychological elements to address with athletes.

Substance Use Disorder

Substance use disorder is a common challenge among athletes and may occur for various reasons. For example, athletes may experience the onset of substance abuse when attempting to cope with career termination (Souter et al., 2018, p. 3). Alternatively, the use of substances or alcohol among athletes can be attributed to social pressures and may even be used to enhance athletic performance in some cases (Gil et al., 2016, p. 1). One example of this includes "doping," which involves using drugs to enhance performance or provide the athlete with a competitive edge (Gil et al., 2016, p. 1). Elite athletes may consume stimulants to enhance their performance, which are highly addictive and may result in physical and psychological dependence with varying tolerance and withdrawal symptoms (Souter et al., 2018, p. 5). Additionally, one study noted that athletes are often exposed to substances at a higher rate than the general population, which increases the opportunity of these individuals to engage in substance misuse (Gil et al., 2016, p. 1). Their need for treatment intervention may, therefore, be higher than that of the general population.

The onset of substance abuse can involve several different substances or the misuse of alcohol, including binge drinking (Souter et al., 2018, p. 5). The role of co-occurring conditions is also commonly associated with the onset of substance misuse, due to beliefs that other interventions will be ineffective or concerns regarding the potential stigmatization of seeking mental health care (Donohue et al., 2016, p. 273). Alternatively, in some cases, the athlete is unaware of their psychological condition or symptoms and uses a substance to cope with the unidentified symptoms (Donohue et al., 2016). Therefore, there is often an underlying and co-occurring disorder that leads to the substance use disorder (Levit et al., 2018, p. 803). Additionally, the presence of injuries and pain can contribute to a substance use condition (Gil et al., 2016, p. 1). It is therefore important to take seriously substance misuse among athletes.

ROLE OF INJURIES IN CO-OCCURRING DISORDERS

Injuries can play a significant role in the development of co-occurring conditions in athletes. Athletic injuries are also common in the United States, with approximately 2 million high school athletes experiencing an injury each year (Gil et al., 2016, p. 5). An athlete that experiences injury will often experience several adjustments in their life, including emotional adjustment, which can be challenging after an injury has occurred (Thompson & Schary, 2020, p. 1). One study noted that the onset of an injury was associated with the development of depression in athletes and the development of co-occurring anxiety (Souter et al., 2018, p. 2). The onset of several mental health conditions has been found in athletes after an injury (Souter et al., 2018, p. 2). These conditions may become co-occurring and cause major challenges for athletes in their future.

Common athletic injuries include those to the head and joint, with head injuries having a major correlation with the onset of depression (Souter et al., 2018, p. 2). Other common injuries can include musculoskeletal injuries and the need to undergo multiple surgeries (Gouttebarge et al., 2019, p. 700). The physical pain from injuries can lead players to engage in forms of "self-treatment" through substance and alcohol misuse, which can create further challenges and co-occurring conditions (Gouttebarge et al., 2019, p. 705). Additionally, much like transition experiences, injuries among athletes may lead to a loss of identity, which has become centered around their athletic ability and performance (Souter et al., 2018, p. 3). Furthermore, though athletes often receive rehabilitation treatments and therapies, they are less likely to receive therapy for their mental health or for the presence of co-occurring conditions that can be created as a result (Gil et al., 2016, p. 1). Injuries may therefore play a large role as gateway drugs for athletes.

COUNSELING AS A VITAL TOOL TO ATHLETES

Counseling should be considered a vital tool for athletes and their overall well-being. In the realm of college education, athletic students experience additional stressors from their non-athletic counterparts as they must maintain peak performance and remain in peak physical condition (Moreland et al., 2018, p. 58). For example, athletes must balance the challenges associated with their sport and performance, while also focusing on obtaining high levels of academic performance and success (Moreland et al., 2018, p. 59). These high-pressure demands often result in the development of mental health conditions that must be effectively addressed (Moreland et al., 2018, p. 58). However, several challenges and barriers often stand in the way of athletes receiving the care required, which must also be addressed.

One option that can be employed among the general athletic population includes well-being therapy (WBT), which assists athletes in engaging in self-observation to identify areas that require strategies to overcome (Thompson & Schary, 2020, p. 2). This approach relies on intrinsic motivation but offers athletes the tools necessary to identify and address challenges as they arise (Thompson & Schary, 2020, p. 3). Moreover, the WBT method involves three important stages of therapy, including self-observation, identification, and cognitive restructuring, which allow for the athlete to reflect on their situation, identify the problem, and use cognitive-behavioral strategies to address them (Thompson & Schary, 2020, p. 5). This is one of many interventions that can be used by athletes to enhance their well-being.

However, it is important to allow for optimization of mental health geared toward athletes that is accompanied by the removal of stigma often associated with its use (Purcell et al., 2019, p. 2). Moreover, it may be beneficial to implement a controlled evaluation system to assist in identifying athletes that require intervention services (Donohue et al., 2016, p. 275). The negative perceptions of mental health care must also be addressed during this process (Donohue et al., 2016, p. 273). Addressing the needs of athletes effectively and in a timely manner may require the use of brief anti-stigma interventions and a clear description of mental health programs that can assist in facilitating a path to therapy while also reducing one of the major barriers to care simultaneously (Purcell et al., 2019, p. 2). Providing mental health care to athletes is an important component to enhancing their well-being and performance, making it a vital tool for athletes in the future.

SUMMARY

The prevalence of co-occurring mental health disorders among athletes is high and often attributed to high levels of stress and standards of perfectionism. These co-occurring mental health conditions involve a variety of mental health challenges, including depression and anxiety disorders, eating and exercise disorders, and the onset of substance use disorder to cope with other conditions. The presence of an athletic injury can increase the risk of developing a mental health disorder or substance use disorder and requires effective intervention methods to decrease its impact or prevent its occurrence. However, the levels of stigma surrounding mental health care stand in the way of it being utilized as a vital tool to assist athletes in these challenging times. The research conducted was eye-opening to the extent that athletes are impacted by pressures, transitions, and injuries overall. The studies explored demonstrate the need to enhance and increase access to care, while also changing the attitudes in society revolving around seeking treatment. Employing therapeutic interventions can be life-changing and assist athletes in overcoming challenges while reducing the risk of developing co-occurring conditions.

DISCUSSION QUESTIONS

The closing of this research project also aims to pose some questions for future discussion.

1. In what ways can social stigmas around mental health care and athletes be addressed?
2. In the future, how does society increase access to mental health services for athletes?
3. Should athletic leaders, including colleges, be responsible for providing mental health care to their athletes?
4. How can conditions such as eating disorders and exercise disorders be effectively addressed when pressures for peak physical condition and performance is required?
5. Can public funding be increased to provide sports-related therapy to those in need to fill the current gap in therapy offerings?

REFERENCES

Donohue, B., Dowd, A., Philips, C., Plant, C. P., Loughran, T., & Gavrilova, Y. (2016). Controlled evaluation of a method to assist recruitment of participants into treatment outcome research and engage student-athletes into substance abuse intervention. *Journal of Clinical Sport Psychology, 10*(4), 272–288. https://doi.org/10.1123/jcsp.2015-0022

Gil, F., De Andrade, A. G., & Castaldelli-Maia, J. M. (2016). Discussing prevalence, impacts, and treatment of substance use disorders in athletes. *International Review of Psychiatry, 28*(6), 572–578. https://doi.org/10.1080/09540261.2016.1212821

Gouttebarge, V., Castaldelli-Maia, J. M., Gorczynski, P., Hainline, B., Hitchcock, M. E., Kerkhoffs, G. M., Rice, S. M., & Reardon, C. L. (2019). Occurrence of mental health symptoms and disorders in current and former elite athletes: A systematic review and meta-analysis. *British Journal of Sports Medicine, 53*(11), 700–706. https://doi.org/10.1136/bjsports-2019-100671

Hauck, C., Schipfer, M., Ellrott, T., & Cook, B. (2020). "Always do your best!"—The relationship between food addiction, exercise dependence, and perfectionism in amateur athletes. *German Journal of Exercise and Sport Research, 50*(1), 114–122. https://doi.org/10.1007/s12662-019-00609-x

Levit, M., Weinstein, A., Weinstein, Y., Tzur-Bitan, D., & Weinstein, A. (2018). A study on the relationship between exercise addiction, abnormal eating attitudes, anxiety and depression among athletes in Israel. *Journal of Behavioral Addictions, 7*(3), 800–805. https://doi.org/10.1556/2006.7.2018.83

Moreland, J. J., Coxe, K. A., & Yang, J. (2018). Collegiate athletes' mental health services utilization: A systematic review of conceptualizations, operationalizations, facilitators, and barriers. *Journal of Sport and Health Science, 7*(1), 58–69. https://doi.org/10.1016/j.jshs.2017.04.009

Purcell, R., Gwyther, K., & Rice, S. M. (2019). Mental health in elite athletes: Increased awareness requires an early intervention framework to respond to athlete needs. *Sports Medicine-Open, 5*(46), 1–8. https://doi.org/10.1186/s40798-019-0220-1

Souter, G., Lewis, R., & Serrant, L. (2018). Men, mental health and elite sport: A narrative review. *Sports Medicine-Open, 4*(57), 1–8. https://doi.org/10.1186/s40798-018-0175-7

Thompson, B. A., & Schary, D. P. (2020). Well-being therapy: An approach to increase athlete well-being and performance. *Journal of Sport Psychology in Action, 12*(1), 1–10. https://doi.org/10.1080/21520704.2020.1750516

Ethics in Sports

INTRODUCTION

Ethics in sports is a double-edged sword. The consequences can become dangerous and even lethal (USADA, 2021). Yet some are skillful enough to know how to reverse the angle of the sword so that that it can be used effectively either way. This chapter will take on a Socratic approach which is controversial, similar to the controversial life of the Greek philosopher who has been termed the father of ethics (Dhillon & Lim, 2015). However, unlike the father of ethics, who did not publish his thoughts, the thoughts in this chapter are delineated to stimulate the rational reasoning that most philosophical minds consider the ultimate objective of ethical thinking. The chapter begins with the question, what is ethics?

WHAT IS MEANT BY ETHICS?

Ethics is sometimes used interchangeably with the concept of morality or moral judgement. However, there is a categorical imperative that suggests a difference in the concepts. Morality or moral judgment is based on a personal foundation of right and wrong or good and bad. For example, children are socialized early in life to believe that they are good or bad based on their behaviors. They are told that they play sports very well and should continue on to become famous. Many of these children grow up motivated to win in sports, to become as famous as the sports idol they adore. They personally spend hours training and conditioning their bodies to perform. But they do not realize something else has to take center court. That is the ethics and ethical issues that will become the greatest nemesis in the sport. Although ethics takes on a less personal aspect, it can either make a career or end a career. Ethics are the rules or principles that are designed to provide uniformity or, as Kant would suggest, a universal imperative that reason alone can guide all individual's behavior in the search for success. Thus, morals or morality is used to make judgments about individuals, whereas ethics is the standard or the road map of how to make choices. Those choices will come with consequences if they are not within the ethical standards of the sport.

Morality is the subjective aspects of personal human behavior that is less formalized and less rigid. Ethics provide the formalized structure that suggests right from wrong in written codes or principles. For example, the NCAA clearly sets standards for athletes and institutions who accept their sponsorship. Therefore, these entities must adhere to the NCAA rules with signed agreements. Socrates may pose the question as to whether it is morally right to have individuals and institutions sign agreements to commit to what is morally right. Further, how or who decides that others are not "fit" to also be part of the sponsorship of the NCAA even if they feel they can morally do what is right and there is no need for a signed agreement? Some athletes and institutions of higher education know goodness and justice, but why act justly if one can profit by doing the opposite (USDOJ, 2019)?

Ethics originated over 2,000 years ago in ancient Greece with Socrates said to be not only the first moral philosopher but also "the greatest philosopher of millennia to come on morality, truth, and virtue" (Dhillon & Lim, 2016, p. 6). Socrates excited his followers, but when more powerful Greek elite governors considered that he had too much attention, he was condemned and executed for his ideas about ethics. He left no writings of his thoughts. His fame and fortune were discredited by rivals. What we know about Socrates's thoughts are primarily from his followers, especially the works of Plato, which is considered the most reliable (Dhillon & Lim, 2015, p. 13). Why is this chapter relevant in a book about sports? The world of sports is based on ethics and moral behavior. Intentionally or unintentionally, every aspect can be explained by ethical theory. Dimmock & Fisher (2017) suggest that there are three branches of ethics: metaethics, normative ethics, and applied ethics.

- Metaethics focuses on what morality is and seeks to understand or find answers to questions. In sports, the metaethicists are sports analysts. They help the audience understand the game and what is going on in the game. They try to make sense of players' behaviors.
- Normative ethics provides the framework for ethics. It tells us how we should live our lives to bring about the best consequences, including conforming to moral laws. In sports games, the referees are the normative ethicists. They interpret the rules and call the fouls when they occur.
- Applied ethics applies the theory to specific issues such as justice, abortion, the death penalty, or animal rights issues. In sports, the applied ethicists are the athletes in the game. They have to figure out how to get the ball, keep the ball, and how to score in order to win the game.

DEALING WITH ETHICAL ISSUES IN SPORTS

The expectation is that most people will do the right thing, understanding that engaging in behaviors that are considered wrong should not be the measure of a "good" person. Children are socialized to believe what is right and what is wrong based on the family belief system. However, that value system may cause conflict when children enter the external world of middle school. At home they were taught not to lie, but in the school sports games, they are told it is okay to say that your foot was not on the line when in fact it was on the line. When children inquire about the confusion, the explanations are typically that it is okay the break the rules in sports because it's only a game; the important thing is to win the game. No one gets hurt. The implication is that "the game" has rules and standards, but it is okay to break them if you don't get caught. Thus, children are socialized to understand that moral values at home about right from wrong are different than those in sports because there are written rules called ethical standards. The message translated is that it is okay to violate some of these standards if they get in the way of winning. There are numerous ethical issues in the world of sports. The focus in this chapter is on three common ethical issues in college: recruitment practices, punishment of athletes, academic integrity of higher education, and doping practices.

Recruitment and Punishment

The literature is replete with information regarding athletic recruitment guidelines and processes (Magnusen et al., 2014). But there is limited information addressing ethical issues related to the recruitment process. They are known and suspected, but either only hinted at or mentioned once in passing (on the news). There does not appear to be an ethical and moral obligation to ensure that all athletes have a fair opportunity to become college or university athletes, and as a result, many of the elite players become victims of ethical violations. NCAA (2021) suggests that recruitment of college athletes can occur with little more than a hello to the potential student and family in the following manner: face-to-face contact, phone, email, text, and social media. Recruitment is observation [termed "evaluation"] of athletes when they are competing with an intentional or unintentional goal of obtaining their services for the betterment of the college or university team. Specific individuals have the responsibility for observing and bringing on new student athletes based on their athletic skills and future potential. Recruiters attend middle and high school games to scout potential candidates. They follow leads provided through social media about high school players.

However, there are rules established by NCAA for recruitment of college athletes. Do all recruiters follow the rules? One rule is that coaches can begin contact with potential recruits in their sophomore year beginning in January 1 of that sophomore year, but recruits should not make official college campus visits until August 1 of their junior year (Frank, 2019). Yet, it is interesting that many athletes have contact and visits during their freshman year. Promises are made to parents, and in some instances, gifts are given to the family. Even though the rule has changed now where college players can earn money with autographs and advertisements, these enticements are presented to athletes and their families before they make scholarship decisions. So the cost of eligibility is no longer threatened by a college athlete accepting external compensation for their athletic ability. This new rule change is said to have a lasting effect on college recruitment because the focus will become how much money can be earned at one institution of higher education versus another institution of higher education (Feather, 2021). Speculations regarding the impact of this change suggest that larger institutions will benefit the most because they will be in a position to offer greater monetary gains to college athletes than smaller or private institutions. Michigan's largest athletic programs have begun to organize their athletic programs to take advantage of this new rule (Feather, 2021). Millions of dollars are spent in the recruitment process for elite athletes. Over a million dollars was reported to have been spent by 21 of the 300 Division I institutions to recruit elite athletes (Sander, 2008), and the number is increasing.

The NCAA has established recruitment guidelines that are specified in the following categories: recruiting terms, campus visits, national letter of intent, Division III Celebratory Signing Form, and recruiting calendars. Even though the NCAA recruiting ethical standards are clearly delineated, the effectiveness of the recruitment process is based primarily on the personal values of the recruiter and the coach (Treadway et al., 2014). Recruiters use many different tactics to recruit elite athletes, including considering school reputation, honeymooning the athlete's family members, discussing future fame and fortune, location, former players, to money and other gifts to entice the athlete to make the decision to attend their school. The ethical concerns occur with recruiting when the recruiter and the coaches cross the NCAA recruiting standards line. For example, Jim Harbaugh, head coach of the Michigan Wolverines, took his team to Florida for what he termed a skill building team trip. In fact, he was taking the team there specifically to recruit elite players from a specific area, giving out his personal telephone number and requesting individuals "reach out" if needed. Coach Harbaugh has also been known to stay at student athlete's homes on recruitment trips (Morgan, 2016).

The Reggie Bush situation is often mentioned in discussions about ethical issues in sports. Bush was a former running back for University of Southern California (USC) who was reported to have received numerous "gifts" (new home, cash, and travel expenses), an NCAA violation for which his Heisman Trophy was taken from him. Because the gifts were presented to Bush by his agent they violated NCAA regulations, and he was severely sanctioned in keeping with NCAA's strong desire to exert and maintain control over student athlete agents (Malinowski, 2019).

When the sports rules are abused or violated, ethical concerns arise. Other areas of ethics involving recruitment include large corporations. Before the new ruling, Adidas executives used cash payments for some universities to obtain elite athletes, which lead to an FBI investigation, arrest, and criminal charges of wire fraud and conspiracy to commit wire fraud for former Adidas executive Jim Gatto (Malinowski, 2019; USDOJ, 2019). Gatto was sentenced to 9 months in federal prison, while Merl Code and Christian Dawkins both received 6 months (Duffy, 2019). University of Louisville coach, Rick Pitino, was given a level 1 sanction by the NCAA: *"failing to promote an atmosphere of compliance"* (Thomson, 2020). After the verdicts were rendered by the federal court, an Adidas company representative made the statement that Adidas strengthened their internal structure and "remains committed to ethical and fair business practices" (James, 2019).

It was this 2017 scandal that forced the NCAA to change the ruling regarding monetary compensation for collegiate athletes. This meant that athletes could hire agents as of April 2019 to represent them for receiving benefits even if they were not drafted professionally. However, the agent must be certified by the NCAA (Malinowski, 2019). The major issue with this ruling is that it specifies male basketball athletes only (excluding females and other sports teams). Also, if the student athlete goes undrafted, they can no longer have an agent–client relationship when the student athlete returns to school. The NCAA's justification is maintaining the amateurism nature of collegiate sports.

Other ethical concerns do not include the sports playing field, but are still relevant to recruitment practices. A diverse management team can help to resolve ethical issues and implement equitable principles that can guide moral and ethical decision-making, external as well as internal to the sports world (Dhillon & Kim, 2016). Dhillon and Kim (2016) suggest that ethics are about honesty, fairness, and trustworthiness. Ethics presumes the need to do what the law requires. Many athletic departments and advisory boards are still patriarchal, comprised of mostly males. In order to seek change in the recruiting process, there will need to be a shift in upper management. More accountability from recruiters and coaches can become a demand from upper management teams. However, this is unlikely to occur with archaic thinking members who have emerged from the ranks of the sports and maintain the same or similar recruiting techniques they were exposed to when they were recruited. Recruitment is a crucial aspect of collegiate sports. We turn now to another component of discussion on ethical behaviors: punishment.

Institutions of higher education are brands and will protect their institutions at any cost, even risking the lives of others on campus (Jacoby, 2019). Federal regulations and guidance around the Family Educational Rights and Privacy Act (FERPA) suggest that information regarding disciplinary administrative hearings that account for a violation of institution rules or policies (that is, punishment/sanctions) can be released to the public. Still, many institutions of higher education do not readily release the information, especially if the student involved happens to be an athlete. The unethical decision to not report athletes' incidents that violate the rules (e.g., hazing, phantom classes, sex assaults) demonstrates what can happen when athletes are not punished for their negative behaviors. When athletic departments do not address and punish behavior, it will continue (USDOJ, 2019).

However, some universities are not able to "get away with" their unethical tactics. For example, in 2016 Baylor University was investigated for a sexual assault scandal involving 19 football players over a 4-year period where sexual allegations of misconduct were not reported. The NCAA investigation focused on allegations that Baylor shielded football student athletes from school disciplinary processes and did not report allegations of misconduct. The university admitted that the allegations were true and noted in a written statement that Baylor University "demand ongoing adherence to ethics and accountability from each and every employee." Baylor's NCAA punishment is a 4-year probation and $5,000 fine. The NCAA noted that the punishment was not severe due to the fact that the Baylor administrators bore much of the responsibility because of a lack of institutional control (a campus-wide culture of nonreporting was pervasive, widespread, and ignored by Baylor's administrators) (Brown, 2021). Although the Department of Education fined Baylor $461,656 for Clery Act violations (not reporting campus crimes between 2011 and 2016), the punishment appears rather interesting. The administrators were allowed to resign, as did football coach Art Briles. The fraternity past president, was given probation, but three of the football student athletes were found guilty and imprisoned, one up to 35 years with probation to be considered only after half of the sentence is served.

Academic Integrity

Academic integrity is an ethical area of major concern, and institutions of higher education may publicly voice concern. However, where athletes are concerned, there appears to be limited attention for reform. Reform is needed in this area to reduce or eliminate the numerous student athletes who play sports, but who may never graduate or who may graduate displaying limited academic skills. Student athletes are isolated either from the main campus or within the main campus in many athletic departments. They have specific advisors assigned to the athletic department and personal tutors who are also typically housed within the athletic department. In some instances, some of their classes are within the athletic department. Athletic directors and coaches have total control over the academic component as well as the sports component. Does this model cause harm? This model can breed illiterate graduates, or it can discourage student athletes from continuing their education. And it can negatively affect the institution because many personnel in the athletic department specialize in sports and not on academic endeavors. Therefore, in their attempts to assist student athletes academically they may utilize "shortcuts" (e.g. plagiarize papers, or use ghost writers). Their focus is to ensure that the student athlete can continue eligibility to win games. These students are being exploited and their futures are of little significance to the institution. The primary concern for the institution is to win games. After all, it is about money.

The NCAA's 14-year 10.8-billion-dollar agreement with television, internet, and wireless rights agreement will be effective from 2014 through 2024. This agreement permits covering of men's basketball Division I championship games (Dyer, 2011). This sacrifice of classroom student success for the sports field or court (Poliakoff & Zhang, 2017) is a model that must be reformed.

Poliakoff and Zhang (2017) provide a clear and striking suggestion for the need to reform with their examples of egregious academic misconduct by Syracuse and the University of North Carolina (UNC) where student athlete class assignments and emails to professors were submitted by ghost writers (members of the athletic department). Ganim and Sayers (2014) revealed a CNN report of 18 years of academic fraudulent behaviors at UNC to ensure that some of their athletes would remain eligible to play. Stanford University's "course of interests list" (considered crème puff classes that anyone can pass) and the University of Michigan's president stating that they admit students who are not academically qualified (Poliakoff & Zhang, 2017) are further instances of institutional academic fraud. These academic integrity issues that are sanctioned by many coaches and institutions of higher education are harmful not only to the student athlete, but also to their families and the community and to future generations who may feel that academics should be second to athletics. The long-term effects of this unethical behavior are not considered. Only a small percentage of the student athletes will enter the professional sports arena. The others will return to their communities still either with only a seventh grade reading and writing competency or totally illiterate (Outlaw, 2019).

Although the NCAA's position on academic fraud is that it is a major violation in Division I sports, the association takes the position of Fletcher's situation ethics (Ridpath et al., 2015), which focus on the purpose served as opposed to cause (Dimmock & Fisher, 2017). Situation ethics suggest that at some time and on some occasions, ethical and moral violations will occur and are acceptable. Thus, academic fraud and misconduct has permeated higher education's quest to bring in millions of dollars through their athletic program, but at the cost, in many instances, of academic integrity and student athletes becoming victims of higher education fraud.

Student athletes' roles expand beyond the dual roles identified in the literature (students and athletes). Their roles are tripled as they struggle with the role of student, the role of athlete, and the extreme struggle for self-identity that places them in a constant battle with ethical issues unlike those nonstudent athletes face. Leaving home to become a student in an academic environment is exciting but scary, and all freshmen experience the journey. Including the athletic component provides not only the protective factors, but risk factors as well, one of which is academic fraud (which some nonathletic students also experience). Personal values may cause conflicting and competing ethical issues for many athletes as they make decisions.

Doping in Collegiate Sports

When the concept "doping" is used, often the image is of illegal drug use becomes the image. But performance-enhancing drugs (PEDs) have been historically an ethical area of concern in sports, dating back to Greek and Roman sports where the use of performance enhancers was acknowledged and condoned (Dandoy & Gereige, 2012; Ekmekci, 2016). Dandoy and Gereige (2012) provide a cursory historical glance at the Roman gladiators who would ingest strychnine in their attempts to prevent injuries while participating in events. It was also thought that strychnine would increase their strength and reduce their levels of fatigue because it provided additional stimulation to the athletes—even though it is a pesticide used to kill rats. However, in the 1960s, PEDs became a major concern in the United States (CNN, 2021). One concern is that when used by athletes in competitive sports, the enhancers are said to provide an unfair advantage over other athletes who are not using enhancers. Enhancers are used by athletes primarily to allow the athlete to perform better than the competitor, to make muscles bigger, to recover faster from injury, and to increase endurance (Mayo Clinic, 2020). Anabolic androgenic steroids are some of the most common PEDs, which reduce body fat and build muscles (NIDA, 2018). Other common PEDs are listed in the table below.

TABLE 10.1 **Classes of Commonly Used Performance-Enhancing Drugs**

Anabolic Agents	Human manufactured male sex hormone testosterone (muscle building). Used to boost performance. Prohibited by WADA.
Anabolic steroids	Natural synthetic substances that build the muscles and allow quick recovery.
Testosterone	A major anabolic steroid that is a sex steroid hormone. A controlled DEA regulated substance that should only be accessed by a medical doctor.
Steroid precursors	Promote lean body mass. Sold over the counter with minimal regulations.
Dehydroepiandrosterone (DHEA)	DHEA supplements improve muscle strength and endurance. It is a steroid hormone. Prohibited in competitive sports.
Androstenedione	A supplement that has been banned by the MLB, NCAA, Olympics, NFL.
Nutritional Supplements	Popular among adolescent athletes. Easily accessible in stores. Little human testing.
Creatine	Popular nutritional supplement with 6th–12th grade levels reporting use. Not recommended for use under age 18, but not prohibited by WADA.
Protein/amino acids	Supplements that may contain substances on the WADA prohibited list.
β-hydroxy β-methylbutyric acid (HMB)	A sports supplement used as an ergogenic aid by bodybuilders for strength, power, and high performance.
Stimulants (such as amphetamines)	Used to increase alertness.
Ephedrine	A stimulant used as an energizer. Banned by NCAA and the International Olympic Committee.
Caffeine/Guarana	Used in beverages and soft drinks. Used for ergogenic effects. Easily accessible.
Human growth hormone (AKA HGH)	Taken to improve strength and endurance. Banned by WADA. Difficult to detect.
Erythropoietin (EPO)	A type of blood doping used for endurance.
Blood doping	Artificially increasing the red blood cells in the body to increase stamina (performance). Banned by the International Olympic Committee.
Diuretics	Drugs used to increase urine flow. Can serve to mask steroid use. On the WADA prohibited drug list.
Actovegin (calf blood extract)	Calf's blood with white blood cells and protein removed. Helps to recover from injury faster. Does not have FDA approval. Although not on the WADA prohibited substance list, it is not approved for sale in the U.S.

Source: Dandoy, C., & Gereige, R. S. (2012). Performance-enhancing drugs. nih.gov

Bramstedt (2007) suggests that fair play in academics and sports is a continuous battle that is too frequently challenged by the notion of performance-enhancing drugs. Coaches and athletes discover many different ways to cheat, and doping has become publicly recognized as the most widely used cheating component of the sports world (Evans et al., 2017). CNN (2021) provides a factual timeline for use and sanctions regarding PEDs in sports.

Timeline[*]

1967—The International Olympic Committee (IOC) establishes a Medical Commission in response to an increase in the usage of performance-enhancing substances.

1981—After American discus thrower Ben Plucknett tests positive for steroids, he is banned from participating in future events by the International Amateur Athletics Federation (IAAF), and he is stripped of his world record.

1987—The National Football League (NFL) begins testing players for steroids.

1988—The U.S. Congress passes the Anti-Drug Abuse Act, which makes possession and distribution of anabolic steroids for nonmedical purposes a crime.

1990—Congress strengthens the 1988 law by classifying anabolic steroids as a controlled substance.

1999—The World Anti-Doping Agency (WADA) is established.

2000—The U.S. Anti-Doping Agency (USADA) is established.

2002—Federal authorities launch an investigation into BALCO, a California lab that is suspected of selling performance-enhancing drugs to athletes.

2003—Major League Baseball (MLB) begins testing players for steroids.

February 2005—Retired baseball star Jose Canseco publishes his autobiography, *Juiced: Wild Times, Rampant 'Roids, Smash Hits and How Baseball Got Big*. In the book, Canseco recounts his own steroid use and implicates other players.

March 2005—Six former and current Major League Baseball players testify before the House Government Reform Committee about drugs in baseball. They include Mark McGwire, Sammy Sosa, and Canseco.

March 2006—MLB Commissioner Bud Selig announces an investigation into steroid use among pro baseball players. Former U.S. Sen. George Mitchell will lead the investigation.

August 22, 2006—The USADA bans sprinter Justin Gatlin for 8 years after he tests positive for banned substances a second time. Gatlin is also forced to forfeit his 100-meter world record.

---

[*] CNN, Selection from "Performance Enhancing Drugs in Sports Fast Facts." https://www.cnn.com/2013/06/06/us/performance-enhancing-drugs-in-sports-fast-facts/index.html. Copyright © 2022 by Cable News Network. Reprinted with permission.

May 2007—1996 Tour de France winner Bjarne Riis admits using performance-enhancing drugs to win his title. Race organizers tell him to return his yellow first-place jersey.

September 20, 2007—Cyclist Floyd Landis is stripped of his 2006 Tour de France title and is banned for 2 years after a positive test for synthetic testosterone.

December 13, 2007—The Mitchell Report is released. MLB players named in the steroid report include Barry Bonds, Roger Clemens, and Andy Pettitte.

February 2008—Former New York Mets clubhouse employee Kirk Radomski is sentenced to 5 years of probation after pleading guilty to distributing steroids.

February 2009—Alex Rodriguez admits to using performance-enhancing drugs while playing for the Texas Rangers.

January 2010—McGwire admits to using steroids during his career.

February 2012—Three-time Tour de France winner Alberto Contador is stripped of his 2010 title for doping.

June 2012—The USADA confirms that it is opening proceedings against Lance Armstrong and five former teammates. Armstrong denies the charges. …

August 2012—American cyclist Tyler Hamilton is stripped of his gold medal from the 2004 Olympics after he admits to doping.

January 2013—MLB announces it will begin random testing for HGH.

July 2013—Ryan Braun of the Milwaukee Brewers is suspended without pay for the remainder of the 2013 season for violating the league's drug policy.

August 2014—Anthony Bosch, the founder of a Miami anti-aging clinic, surrenders to the Drug Enforcement Administration. He later pleads guilty to a charge of distributing steroids to athletes. His sentence is 4 years in federal prison.

September 2014—The NFL and NFL Players Association reach an agreement regarding the league's performance-enhancing drug policy. The agreement calls for HGH testing and an overhaul of the drug program.

January 2015—Kenya's Rita Jeptoo, a three-time Boston Marathon champion, is banned from competition for 2 years for doping.

September 2015—The DEA announces that 90 people have been arrested and 16 underground steroid labs have been shut down in a sweeping drug bust called Operation Cyber Juice.

November 9, 2015—A WADA report details evidence of doping in Russian athletics and a "deeply rooted culture of cheating at all levels." Russia is later provisionally suspended as a member of the International Association of Athletics Federations.

March 2016—At a press conference, tennis player Maria Sharapova admits to failing a drug test at the Australian Open. She is initially suspended for 2 years, but the ban is later reduced to 15 months.

July 18, 2016—A WADA report alleges Russia ran a state-sponsored doping program during the 2014 Sochi Winter Olympics. On December 9, 2016, WADA releases an update to the report concluding that a "systematic and centralized cover-up" benefited more than 1,000 Russian athletes across 30 sports.

August 4, 2016—The IOC announces that 271 athletes from the 389-member Russian Olympic team have been cleared to participate in the 2016 Rio Olympics. The rest of the team—118 athletes—are banned in the wake of the doping scandal.

August 7, 2016—A swimmer from the Chinese Olympic team tests positive for a banned substance called hydrochlorothiazide, a blood pressure drug that doubles as a diuretic.

August 11, 2016—John Anzrah, a sprint coach for the Kenyan Olympic team, is sent home after allegedly posing as an athlete to take a drug test. He is the second Kenyan running coach to face allegations that he tried to help athletes cheat on doping tests. Michael Rotich, the team's track and field manager, reportedly tried to bribe undercover journalists posing as coaches, offering to pay them in exchange for advance warning about drug tests.

August 24, 2016—The International Weightlifting Federation reports that 15 Olympic weight lifters, including three Chinese gold medalists, have tested positive for illegal growth hormones and other banned substances in doping retests.

January 25, 2017—The IOC rules that Usain Bolt's 2008 gold medal in the 4x100m relay no longer counts after one of his teammates tests positive for methylhexaneamine, a banned substance.

June 29, 2017—Michelle Payne, a Melbourne Cup winning jockey, is banned from competing for 4 weeks after failing a drug test.

December 5, 2017—The IOC announces that Russia is banned from the 2018 Winter Olympics in South Korea because of the country's "systematic manipulation" of anti-doping rules. However, Russian athletes who can prove that they are clean will be "invited" to compete. The ban is the most wide-ranging punishment ever meted out by the IOC on a participating country. Russia's Olympic Committee is also ordered to reimburse the IOC $15 million for the cost of the investigation and to help establish a new independent testing authority.

February 1, 2018—The Court of Arbitration for Sport (CAS) overturns lifetime bans on 28 Russian athletes accused of doping, making them eligible to compete in the 2018 Winter Olympics. In 11 additional cases, the athletes are suspended from participating in the 2018 Winter Olympics but they are cleared to compete in future events as the court rules that lifetime bans were not justified.

February 9–25, 2018—The IOC allows 169 Russian athletes to participate in the 2018 Winter Olympics. They are not members of a Russian team. Instead, each participant is called an "Olympic athlete from Russia." They do not carry the Russian flag or wear uniforms that identify them as Russian. Their medals are not added to the country's Olympic medal count.

February 28, 2018—The IOC announces that it is lifting the suspension on Russia participating in the Olympics. The country's status is restored after investigators confirm that there were no additional doping violations by Russian athletes who competed in the 2018 Winter Olympics.

December 9, 2019—WADA unanimously agrees to ban Russia from major international sporting competitions—notably the Olympics and the World Cup—for 4 years over doping noncompliance. On December 17, 2020, CAS reduces the ban to 2 years.

March 9, 2020—Federal prosecutors announce more than 24 people involved in the horse racing industry have been indicted for taking part in a scheme to give racehorses performance-enhancing drugs to help them win races around the world. One of the defendants is trainer Jason Servis, who prosecutors say "doped virtually all horses under his control," including Maximum Security, the colt that crossed the finish line first in the 2019 Kentucky Derby but was disqualified for interference.

March 12, 2021—The UK's Medical Practitioners Tribunal Service (MPTS) finds that former British Cycling and Team Sky doctor Richard Freeman is guilty of ordering testosterone "knowing or believing it was to be administered to an athlete to improve their athletic performance." Following the MPTS decision, UK Anti-Doping (UKAD) has placed Dr. Freeman on "a provisional suspension from all sport."

May 1, 2021—Medina Spirit wins the 147th running of the Kentucky Derby. Just over a week later, Hall of Fame trainer Bob Baffert reveals the 3-year-old colt tested positive for elevated levels of betamethasone, an anti-inflammatory corticosteroid sometimes used to relieve joint pain in horses, throwing Medina Spirit's victory into question.

February 8, 2022—It is announced that 15-year-old Kamila Valieva, a member of the ROC figure skating team, tested positive for a banned substance. Valieva is provisionally suspended but on February 14, the Court of Arbitration for Sports rules she is able to compete in the women's single skating short program event and the women's single skating free skating event at the Beijing Olympics.

Due to systemic doping (use of PEDs) charges detected in Russian athletes, Russia has been suspended from participation in the next two Olympic Games and will have to pay the World Anti-Doping Agency (WADA) $1.27 million for their investigation of the doping by the Russian athletes. The suspension ends December 16, 2022 (Wamsley & Kennedy, 2020). Russia's noncompliance to international anti-doping rules and regulations suggests that although the country received the suspension, athletes from the country will still be able to participate in sports, but not under the country's flag or uniform. What message is this sending to young athletes aspiring to become future Olympians? The United States Anti-Doping Agency (USADA) indicated disappointment with the decision, stating that WADA and clean athletes received a loss in this situation (Wamsley & Kennedy, 2020) and it will be difficult to regain losses as the decision regarding Russian's noncompliance was based on political entities as opposed to ethical reasoning.

The use of PEDs continues as a major ethical concern also because the age of the individuals in sports using the drugs are decreasing, with younger children using PEDs (Dandoy & Gereige, 2012). Even with the establishment of the World Anti-Doping Agency in 1999, there has been no decrease in the use of PEDs. This agency was formed in Switzerland with the mission of creating a drug-free sports environment with their identified core values as (a) protecting the rights of athletes, (b) observing the highest ethical standards, and (c) developing policies and procedures that reflect justice, equity, and integrity (WADA, 2021). A year later the United States developed the USADA. However, its focus appears to be research (USADA, 2021). With headquarters in Colorado, the USADA becomes involved in investigative issues related to drug use among athletes. Although these agencies could possibly be positive entities in the sports environment, there does not appear to be coordinated efforts to establish their missions. And since the formation of the agencies, there does not appear to have been a reduction in the use of PEDs among athletes, but instead there appears to have been an increase in the number of younger children using PEDs. In addition, designer steroids are a particularly dangerous class of anabolic steroids that are undetectable and designed specifically for athletes. These designer steroids have not received FDA approval, nor have they been clinically tested (Mayo Clinic, 2020). Similar to other designer drugs, designer steroids may be impure, mislabeled, and cause instant death due to unknown ingredients.

Why Dope?

Why would so many promising young athletes use PEDs when they know that they are prohibited? Why do coaches and training personnel encourage or close a blind eye to young athletes who engage in doping? Research and personal accounts have provided the answers to these questions. Young collegiate athletes do it to fit in because they see teammates do it. Some want to become the best and view PEDs as the best option for accomplishing their goal. Others want to heal fast from an injury so that they can continue to play their sport. And imagine attempting to maintain the image of elite athlete and continue the expected outstanding performances in every game, not wanting to disappoint fans, family, or the coach. The coach and trainers, on the other hand, have different reasons for encouraging PEDs because they want the athlete to perform at the highest level possible whether injured or healthy. The student athlete's performance determines the coach's salary and further negotiations for incentive bonuses. Berkowitz (2022) reported that despite the pandemic, 21 U.S. college coaches will earn at least 5 million dollars this season. Nick Saban of the University of Alabama is the highest paid at $9,753,221 and Ed Orgeron of Louisiana State University is in second place at $9,012,917. Thus, it is no surprise that even though doping can harm student athletes physically and mentally and can harm their future careers, coaches make unethical decisions about their student athletes and PEDs. Safety and ethical issues become minor considerations for student athletes when million-dollar salaries are at stake.

Many of these coaches function under what they consider the sport ethic, which is based on values and norms defined by team membership for athletes (Ford, Masters, & Vosloo, 2022). Ford et al. (2022) provide an interesting paradigm on doping that can be related to this discussion about coaches' salaries and how they rationalize the limited or lack of protection of their athletes from doping (PEDs). Coaches use the sport ethic to justify their behavior. The sport ethic according to Ford et al. (2022) is composed of the following four components:

- student athletes must be dedicated to the game above all else in their lives;
- student athletes must strive for distinction, which is maintained in an isolated environment in order to instill the notion of winning as a top priority;

- student athletes must understand and accept the risks that are involved in sports, must have no fear of injury, and must demonstrate an ability to perform even when injured; and
- student athletes should not allow anything or anyone to deter them from accomplishing the goal.

Based on this sport ethic, it is reasonable, according to the coach and the student athlete, to use a prohibited drug or even an illegal drug because the sport ethic is greater than the values that were instilled in the student athlete before entering higher education. In many of the social sciences, behavior is grounded in theory. Thus, the Ford et al. (2022) sport ethic is grounded in what they term "positive deviance," which is considered an over conformity to social norms. Hughes and Coakley's (1991) thinking regarding over conformity is what makes student athletes use PEDS. The student athlete does not want only to be a "good" sports athlete, but there is the need to be the *best*, based on the sport ethic that is drilled into them daily by coaches and coaching staff. They normalize injury and pain and consider the lack of ability to compete in their sport as letting the coach and the team down. The inability to compete would be a threat to their identify as a "real" athlete (Hughes & Coakley, 1991, p. 308). It is the sport ethic that distinguishes the real athlete from others.

Consequences for Using PEDs

Unfortunately, the use of PEDs is a common practice now to advance athletic performance (Mayo Clinic, 2020). However, the risks for taking such a dangerous step simply to win seem rather extreme because the consequences can be lethal (USADA, 2021). If an athlete is an undetected PEDs user, that athlete is likely to receive numerous honors and awards. The athlete who is discovered as a PEDs user, may not receive honors and awards, but the aftermath may be the same for both the detected PEDs abuser and the undetected PEDs user. They both face risky side effects if abusing PEDs, including high blood pressure, cancer, stroke, blood clots, and lack of mental well-being.

Some legal consequences of using PEDs are exemplified in the sanctions imposed by WADA on Russia, such as being stripped of metals, prize money forfeited and the country represented may have to pay money for the investigation, and the country's participation in International and national sports can be suspended, and disqualification of all standing records. In the situation of collegiate athletes, as in the case of Reggie Bush, the Heisman trophy can be forfeited as well as loss of scholarship and federal penalties can also be imposed.

It has been difficult to detect and punish athletes who use substances that have been prohibited because of micro doping, which is taking small doses of a drug over a couple of days (Lembo & Naftulin, 2021). The thinking is that if smaller amounts are taken by the time the sport event is finished, the substance will not be detected in blood or urine. As athletes and coaches consider methods for deceiving PEDs detectors, researchers and scientists are also considering the use of technology to improve PEDs detection. The Nanobiosensors is considered a tool that can be used to enhance doping detection by providing greater sensitivity and live-time monitoring (Evans et al., 2017).

Nanosensors

Technology has completely engulfed the world. The impact on the sport world is constantly evolving, revolutionizing the game, and forcing abusers of PEDs to become more creative. A nanosensor is a sensing device used to obtain information and convert the information into data that is analyzed (Javaid et al.,

2021). Nanotechnology is becoming a norm in sports. Nanotechnology was first used and identified by Japanese scientist Norio Taniguchi in 1974. This technology is used to detect and monitor physical and chemical properties at the nano site (Javaid et al., 2021). In the sport world, nanobiosensors will be used for monitoring, training, and competition purposes. The overall aim of the nanobiosensors is to ensure clean competition among athletes; however, the parameters for safe use by athletes have not been clearly delineated (Evans et al., 2017). The nanobiosensors can be used to detect abuse of PEDs by testing urine and ingesting.

One of the major areas of concern regarding ethical issues related to the use of nanobiosensors is that they must be programmed. This poses the question about the programmers and their intent. For example, nanobiosensors can be programmed to harm another athlete by impeding an athletic performance (Evans et al., 2017). There should be policy and procedures designed and implemented to ensure clarity of the process.

Nanotechnological products are also used for other measures. HQ Inc. developed a pill that helps monitor the athlete's body temperature, which is effective when training in hot weather as a means of avoiding heat strokes. This sensor is currently being used by some professional teams (Sehadri et al., 2019). This monitor provides useful training data but also acts as a deterrent to alert the athlete and coaches to potential heat strokes. The Kanaan Company has developed a sensor shirt (sensors embedded within the material) to provide data on the athlete wearing the shirt. The NFL players association has approved a fitness tracker wristband for its players. This wristband tracks physical data and sleep data using five sensors that measure data 100 times per second. The data is automatically transmitted to the WHOOP mobile and Web Apps for analyses and actionable recommendations. In this instance, the players of the players association bargained to own their data. The wristbands cannot be used during competition with other teams.

Due to the serious nature of the use of PEDs in sports, the World Health Organization has identified the recreational use of PEDs as a public health issue, with the physical and psychological effects well established (Smith et al., 2021). Family physicians have an ethical responsibility to ensure that medical intervention and prevention strategies focus on a holistic model of practice. This implies that screening questions should also include questions regarding nutritional supplements and other PEDs. Collegiate involvement in sports is a risk factor as dual roles of student and athlete place the athlete at high risk for PEDs abuse or misuse (Ford et al., 2022). Medical doctors should be aware of the ethical guidelines involved when treating athletes. The same medical standards that apply to the general application of medical knowledge should also apply when treating athletes in sports and exercise medicine.

The physician's role raises numerous questions in the anti-doping discussions, such as physician–client relationship, confidentiality and privacy issues, and justice and fairness (Ekmekci, 2016). Physicians are caught in an ethical dilemma because they are to do no harm to patients according to their Hippocratic Oath, yet when repairing injured athletes, there may be a need to use PEDs for quick recovery and increased patient stamina. However, then goal is not for performance enhancement or advancement, but for the well-being of the patient. The line really becomes an ethical dilemma for the physician if the student athlete is injured during competition and the best medical choice is a drug on the prohibited list of drugs. Another ethical major area of concern for physicians working with student athletes is the issue of confidentiality and privacy. Does a coach or trainers have the right to know the athlete's medical condition? The argument may be that they do have a right in order to address the medical issue with care when the athlete returns for play. How much medical information is too much, and how much is too little for athletes?

SUMMARY

Ethical arguments against doping have included subjects of academic cheating, cheating on the playing field/court, and harm to athletes, coaches, institutions of higher learning, families, and the community. Consideration should also be given to ethical issues in the medical profession—those who provide medical treatment to student athletes. Unethical behavior in the world of intercollegiate sports does astronomical amounts of harm. In addition, PEDs are affecting young middle school athletes to collegiate elite athletes to the assignment of board members of governing bodies. When working with athletes, it is extremely important to raise questions regarding the use of PEDs. Based on current evidence in the literature, athletes who participate in football, basketball, gymnastics, and weight training are at greater risk for using PEDs (Dandoy & Gereige, 2012). With further exploration through continuous research, more attention can be given to the need for moral and ethical conduct in sports.

Although the World Anti-Doping Agency and the United States Anti-Doping Agency (USADA) focus on the need to create a fair and natural sports environment for athletes, there has been no—or very limited—intention to focus on academic integrity from institutions of higher education. Thus, it still appears that even as ethical issues permeate discussions about elite institutions of higher education and their athletes, this area of concern has not resulted in establishing a worldwide or a U.S. agency to promote similar core values as described by the anti-doping agencies. Academic performance has a lesser role than athletic performance, as demonstrated by the creation of anti-doping agencies. Until we advocate to ensure student athletes' rights to an education equal to their nonathletic peers, and until policies and procedures reflect justice, equity, and integrity for student athletes, the positive deviance will continue to invade the halls of academia and the doping will continue. The important question is, what role will you play in bringing about positive change?

Although Nietzsche suggests that there is no God, it is difficult to refute the notion that there is a need for ethical behavior in sports. This multibillion-dollar world impacts every aspect of social life in American society from the innocent housewife who places her bet on Ohio State University to win another championship game to the organized crime syndicate controlling bets in Las Vegas. It is easy to decide to overlook unethical behaviors by recruiters, coaches, and institutions of higher education; however, these entities are the mentoring features that set the pace for children and future generations. If unethical behaviors continue to be sanctioned for the love of the game or the love of the athlete, what message is passed to future generations? Is the message for them that it is okay to violate rules and standards and laws as long as you profit and can get away with it?

DISCUSSION QUESTIONS

1. In a group, discuss what is meant by ethical dilemma and provide some examples of ethical dilemmas in collegiate sports. Then provide a strategy for how to overcome the dilemma.
2. Identify some current issues related to ethics in collegiate sports. Explain your thoughts providing rationale for why you think the issue emerged. What were the motivating factors that created the ethical issue(s)?
3. Technology is a powerful tool. Provide an example of an advantage and a disadvantage of the use of technology for athlete recruiting purposes.
4. In a group discuss, some issues related to confidentiality when counseling or working with collegiate athletes. How can the issues be overcome? How is HIPAA related this discussion?
5. Using the internet, locate at least two institutions of higher learning that have been involved in unethical athletic practices. How were the situations resolved? Do you think that the sanctions were harsh enough to eliminate future unethical behavior? What sanctions would you have imposed?
6. What are your thoughts about the new NCAA rule (collegiate athletes can now receive external monetary compensation)? What are some advantages and disadvantages to the ruling?

REFERENCES

Berkowitz, S. (2022). Jim Harbaugh said his bonus money would go to Michigan athletes' employees. *USA Today*. https://www.usatoday.com/story/sports/ncaaf/bigten/2022/06/09/michigan-coach-jim-harbaugh-gave-bonus-money-athletics-employees/7559996001/?gnt-cfr=1

Bramstedt, K. A. (2007). Caffeine use by children: The quest for enhancement. *Substance Use & Misuse, 42*(8), 1237–1251. doi: 10.1080/10826080701208962

Brown, D. (2021, August 11). NCAA: Failure to report sexual assault was part of "campus-wide culture of nonreporting" at BU; Briles cleared, attorney says. *KWTX Channel 10 News Report*. https://www.kwtx.com/2021/08/11/ncaa-releases-results-investigation-sparked-by-2016-baylor-sexual-assault-scandal/

CNN. (2021). Performance enhancing drugs in sports fast facts. https://www.cnn.com/2013/06/06/us/performance-enhancing-drugs-in-sports-fast-facts

Dandoy, C., & Gereige, R. S. (2012, June). Performance-enhancing drugs. *Pediatrics in Review, 33*(6), 265–272. https://doi.org/10.1542/pir.33-6-265

Dhillon, N., & Lim, J. (2016). *The greatest Greek philosophers Socrates: The father of ethics & inquiry.* The Rosen Publishing Group, Inc.

Dimmock, R., & Fisher, A. (2017). *Ethics for A-level.* Open Book Publishers. https://books.openbookpublishers.com/10.11647/obp.0125/ch5.xhtml

Duffy, C. (2019). Former Adidas executive gets nine months in jail. *Portland Business Journal.* Sports Business. (bizjournals.com)

Ekmekci, P. E. (2016). Physicians' ethical dilemmas in the context of anti-doping practices. *Annals of Sports Medicine and Research, 3*(7), 1089. https://www.ncbi.nlm.nih.gov/pmc/articles/PMC5215887/

Evans, R., McNamee, M., & Guy, O. (2017). Ethics, nanobiosensors and elite sport: The need for a new governance framework. *Science and Engineering Ethics, 23*, 1487–1505. https://doi.org/10.1007/s11948-016-9855-1

Feather, A. (2021). New NCAA rule could change recruiting forever and provide new opportunities for athletes. *News Channel 3.* https://wwmt.com/news/local/new-ncaa-rule-could-change-recruiting-forever-and-provide-new-opportunities-for-athletes

Ford, J. L., Masters, S., & Vosloo, J. (2022). High school coaches' attitudes toward sport psychology consultation and the barriers to implementation of sport psychology services. *International Journal of Sports Science & Coaching, 17*(5), 999–1008.

Frank, D. (2019). New NCAA DI recruiting rules on early recruiting. NCSA. https://www.ncsasports.org/blog/2019/04/26/ncaa-di-recruiting-rules-early-recruiting/

Ganim, S., & Sayers, D. (2014, October 23). UNC report finds 18 years of academic fraud to keep athletes playing. *CNN Investigations.* https://www.cnn.com/2014/10/22/us/unc-report-academic-fraud

Hughes, R., & Coakley, J. (1991). Positive deviance among athletes: The implications of overconformity to the sport ethic. *Sociology of Sport Journal, 8*(4), 307–325. https://journals.humankinetics.com/view/journals/ssj/8/4/article-p307.xml

Jacoby, J. (2019). College athletes more likely to be disciplined for sex assault. *USA Today.* (usatoday.com)

James, J. (2019). Ex-Adidas worker Jim Gatto to pay over 300K to Kansas, NC State. Coaching Carousel Updates. 247sports.com

Javaid, M., Haleem, A., Singh, R. P., Rab, S., & Suman, R. (2021). Exploring the potential of nanosensors: A brief overview. *Sensors International, 2*, 100130. https://reader.elsevier.com/reader/sd/pii/S2666351121000516?token=8C2FCC51FB40284AF179EF669E3A925A4F173E44AA41624D30331D56AD4258F62B9EBB2A7FA80E1530AECEB4A50828A0&originRegion=us-east-1&originCreation=20211227042122

Lembo, A., & Naftulin, J. (2021, April 30). Everything you need to know about microdosing. *Insider, Inc.* https://www.insider.com/what-is-microdosing-2019-1

Magnusen, M. J., Kim, Y., Perrewe, P. L., & Ferris, G. R. (2014). A critical review and synthesis of student-athlete college choice factors: Recruiting effectiveness in NCAA sports. *International Journal of Sports Science & Coaching, 9*(6), 1265–1266. https://doi.org/10.1260/1747-9541.9.6.1265 https://journals.sagepub.com/doi/10.1260/1747-9541.9.6.1265#

Malinowski, A. (2019). The Adidas college basketball scandal and its aftermath. *Marquette Sports Law Review, 30*(1), 243–263. https://scholarship.law.marquette.edu/cgi/viewcontent.cgi?article=1770&context=sportslaw

Mayo Clinic Staff. (2020). Performance enhancing drugs and teen athletes. The Mayo Clinic. Mayo Foundation for Medical Education and Research (MFMER). Retrieved from: https://www.mayoclinic.org/healthy-lifestyle/fitness/in-depth/performance-enhancing-drugs/art-20046134

McCabe, S. E., West, B. T., Strobbe, S., & Boyd, C. J. (2018). Persistence/recurrence of and remission from DSM-5 substance use disorders in the United States: Substance-specific and substance-aggregated correlates. *Journal of Substance Abuse Treatment, 93*, 38–48.

Morgan, T. (2016). Jim Harbaugh's recruiting methods unethical, irresponsible. *The Record.* https://buffstaterecord.com/6599/sports/jim-harbaughs-recruiting-methods-unethical-irresponsible/

NCAA. (2021). Recruiting-eligibility center. https://www.ncaa.org/student-athletes/future/recruiting

NIDA. (2018, August 12). Anabolic steroids drug facts. National Institutes of Health. https://nida.nih.gov/publications/research-reports/steroids-other-appearance-performance-enhancing-drugs-apeds/how-are-anabolic-steroids-used

Outlaw, K. (2019, December). *Exploring the challenges of elite African American male athletes at predominantly White universities: Three descriptive case studies* (Doctoral dissertation, East Carolina University). http://hdl.handle.net/10342/76170

Poliakoff, M. B., & Zhang, A. (2017, March 13). The ugly truth of March madness. *U.S. News & World Report.* https://www.usnews.com/opinion/op-ed/articles/2017-03-13/march-madness-spotlights-problem-of-academic-integrity-in-college-sports

Ridpath, B. D., Gurney, G., & Snyder, E. (2015). NCAA academic fraud cases and historical consistency: A comparative content analysis. *Journal of Legal Aspects of Sport, 25*(2), 75–103. http://dx.doi.org/10.1123/jlas.2014-0021

Sander, L. (2008, August 1). Have money, will travel: The quest for top athletes. *The Chronicle of Higher Education.* https://www.chronicle.com/article/have-money-will-travel-the-quest-for-top-athletes/

Smith, T., Fedoruk, M., & Eichner, A. (2021). Performance-enhancing drug use in recreational athletes. *American Family Physician, 103*(4), 203–204. https://www.aafp.org/afp/2021/0215/p203.html

Thomson, J. (2020). Men's basketball: Rick Pitino charged with NCAA violation, could face punishment. *Rockland/Westchester Journal News.* https://www.lohud.com/story/sports/college/iona/2020/05/04/ionas-rick-pitino-charged-ncaa-violation-suspension-possible/3079115001/

Treadway, D. C., Adams, G., Hanes, T. J., Perrewé, P. L., Magnusen, M. J., & Ferris, G. R. (2014). The roles of recruiter political skill and performance resource leveraging in NCAA football recruitment effectiveness. *Journal of Management, 40*(6), 1607–1626. https://doi.org/10.1177/0149206312441836; https://journals.sagepub.com/doi/abs/10.1177/0149206312441836

USADA. (2021). Effects of performance enhancing drugs. https://www.usada.org/athletes/substances/effects-of-performance-enhancing-drugs/

USDOJ. (2019). Former Adidas executive, former Adidas consultant, and aspiring manager all sentenced to prison terms for their roles in defrauding Adidas-sponsored NCAA Division I universities. https://www.justice.gov/usao-sdny/pr/former-adidas-executive-former-adidas-consultant-and-aspiring-manager-all-sentenced

Wamsley, L., & Kennedy, M. (2020). Russia gets its doping ban reduced but will miss next 2 Olympics. *NPR News.* https://www.npr.org/2020/12/17/947504052/russia-suspended-from-next-2-olympic-games-over-anti-doping-violations

World Anti-Doping Agency (WADA). (2021). *World Anti-Doping code.* https://www.wada-ama.org/sites/default/files/resources/files/2021_wada_code.pdf

Drug Use by Sport Subculture

INTRODUCTION

The use of performance-enhancing drugs in professional sports has been the subject of intense controversy and scandal in recent years (Weber, 2014). For example, major league baseball has been rocked to its very foundations by scandals over steroids and other performance-enhancing drugs (p. 274). These scandals raised serious questions about the integrity of admired, well-paid players, and even about the professional future of the great American pastime. Weber (2014) states, "At this point, however, the problem of PEDs greatly threatens the health of baseball players and diminishes the continued integrity, popularity, and economic success of baseball" (p. 270). The despair felt within the baseball community and among the players is felt throughout many sports, both professional and amateur alike. Even in youth sports, the pressure to be bigger, faster, and stronger is driving some athletes to look to drugs to enhance their performance, if only to be able to contend on a level playing field. Drug use in sports is a prolific problem—and one for which no particular sport has come up with a solution.

DRUGS IN SPORTS

Juiced

The professional baseball controversy was already raging when Jose Canseco (2005) released his book *Juiced*, which discussed various aspects of his stellar career and candidly described his illegal use of anabolic steroids and human growth hormone to enhance his performance. Indeed, the book indicated that Canseco had used performance-enhancing drugs almost throughout his entire 16-year-long career in the league, from his very first season in 1988 to his final year in 2001 (Canseco, 2005). Thus, it emerged that illegal performance-enhancing drugs had played dominant roles in a career marked by such spectacular high points as 42 home runs and 40 stolen bases in 1988 (Canseco, 2005). *Juiced* was also devastating for its author's allegations of the pervasive use of readily available steroids in Major League Baseball. Canseco actually listed the names of a number of beloved players, including Mark McGwire, Juan Gonzalez, Ivan Rodriguez, and Rafael Palmeiro, whom he claimed had also relied on steroids and other drugs. Indeed, Canseco alleged that he had taught many of these players how to use steroids, and that he even injected some of them with the drugs himself (Canseco, 2005).

Quite apart from the negative side effects associated with many performance-enhancing drugs, reliance on such drugs in professional sports also raises serious questions about fairness and ethical conduct. The major problem rests in the fact that these drugs render their users artificially superior, giving them unfair advantages compared with more honest competitors whose performance relies mainly on genetics, discipline, and hard training (Murray, 2018). This may be the case, for instance, when professional bodybuilders and other professional athletes use creatine to appear more "bulked up" prior to a competition (Sanchez-Oliver et al., 2019). Because much of the perceived muscle bulk would actually be due to the shifting of water to the muscles, an athlete might gain credit for an appearance that is not due to actual muscle mass or real strength. In effect, therefore, an athlete who abused a drug in this manner would be relying upon deception, presenting bodies or performances that leave the impression they were honed and developed through greater dedication, sacrifice, and hard work than the athlete was willing to undertake. At the same time, those ethical athletes who did not rely on such drugs would be placed at a significant disadvantage in competition (Sanchez-Oliver et al., 2019; Weber, 2014). Thus, the use of performance-enhancing drugs by some professional athletes exerts pressures upon others to engage in similar unethical behaviors in order to compensate for the unfair advantages against them (Murray, 2018). As the abuse of performance-enhancing drugs becomes increasingly widespread within a professional sport, individual athletes are all pressured to rely on such drugs in order to stop themselves from lagging behind the rest of the field.

Recently, government regulators, including the Federal Trade Commission, are attempting to protect both athletes and consumers against the dangers associated with PEDs (Silverberg, 2010). Their first concern is the lack of disclosure regarding possible risks. Sports medicine physicians share a secondary concern with the FTC. Too little is known about the stimulant supplements being used by athletes. Worse, many athletes assume that if a little of the product is good, then more of it is better.

Performance-Enhancing Drugs

The abuse of performance-enhancing drugs by influential, tend-setting professional athletes encourages other aspiring athletes to do the same (Murray, 2018; Weber, 2014). Many young athletes look up to their professional sports heroes as role models whose performances and behaviors set the standards to which they aspire. In fact, the abuse of anabolic steroids among many professional athletes exerts intense pressures on young kids to build greatly more muscular bodies, which they frustratingly find are only possible to achieve with drugs. Recent investigations have revealed troubling increases in the reliance on performance-enhancing drugs among ever-younger athletes (Murray, 2018). For example, Chirico et al. (2021) report that while it is commonly supposed that reliance on such drugs is a phenomenon confined mainly to high-performing professional athletes, evidence indicates that disturbing numbers of young American students are abusing performance-enhancing drugs at the high school, junior high school, and even middle school levels. Specialists in the field are highly alarmed by abuse of these potentially dangerous drugs at such young ages, particularly because the overwhelming majority of the medical and scientific investigations into the impacts of performance-enhancing drugs on humans have focused on adult subjects (Chirico et al., 2021). In this respect, the abuse of performance-enhancing drugs by professional athletes seriously undermines the spirits of sportsmanship upon which both professional and amateur sports should be based and potentially endangers the health and well-being of ever-younger athletes (Chirico et al., 2021; Murray, 2018).

Regulation?

Unfortunately, although American society typically places strong faith in the ability of stricter regulations and laws and harsher penalties to resolve critical problems that are ethical in nature at their roots, some evidence suggests that such heavy emphasis on legality might not be adequate for ensuring the truly ethical conduct that the sporting world so desperately needs. Indeed, there are some reasons for believing that more rigid regulations might actually serve to undermine illegal behavior over the long term (Weber, 2014). Analysis from the business world suggests that as regulations and legislations become stricter and more severe, many professionals come to rely less on ethical standards as their guides for conduct and behavior, becoming more concerned with ensuring compliance with rules and laws (Weber, 2014). This often leads in turn for a search for regulatory or legal loopholes and encourages professionals to feel that their behaviors are entirely acceptable, providing they do not overstep the boundaries established by the rules and laws, even though there is often some difference between what is legal and what is ethical (Weber, 2014). In addition, because compliance with even more rigid rules and laws exerts pressures on professional bottom lines, players in a field are pressured to resort to whatever is permissible by the regulations or legislations in order to boost their competitive edges. Conduct is therefore steadily pushed beyond ethical limits in an effort to maintain and increase one's profits (Weber, 2014). As behaviors become ever more egregious, regulations are tempted to step in yet again to implement even stricter rules and laws, thereby creating more bottom-line pressures and perpetuating a vicious, seemingly unending cycle (Weber, 2014).

Olympics

One significant example of an area of sports that have been adversely affected by the influence of PEDs is the Olympics. The Olympic games have been hugely impacted by athletes' drive for perfection. The use of drugs to increase performance at the games can be traced to the third century BC (Rosen, 2008). Both national and international sports federations ban a variety of drugs and doping techniques in elite sports. The concern is not about the safety of the athletes. The rules were designed to protect all athletes from the unfair advantage gained by the few athletes who use substances to improve their performance. With legal stimulants used in mass quantities in the United States in the form of caffeine, appetite suppressants, or decongestants, it is difficult to draw the line between appropriate and excessive use. It is understandable that an athlete would turn to drugs to improve performance, similar to how most of society turns to drugs to alleviate a physical inconvenience. But this excuse does not justify the athlete who uses stimulants illegally.

SUMMARY

What would seem to be needed, therefore, is not an overemphasis on stricter regulations and laws and more severe punishments, but also an increased focus on ethics. Though there is clearly a need for improved rules and laws in cases where serious abuses are possible, the nation also needs to have a serious, frank discussion about the ethical state of its society. One simply cannot expect that rules and laws will lead to ethical conduct and behavior. Nor can one hope to effect real change with discussions that focus solely on professional sportsmen and women. After all, the recent spectacular scandals at several highly respected American companies demonstrate that the problem of cheating is hardly confined to doping among professional athletes. One can hardly expect sporting professionals and aspiring young athletes to aim for the ethical high road when the rest of society appears to be aiming for significantly lower goals.

One can easily understand why athletes would choose to use drugs to enhance their performance, particularly within a society such as the United States, in which pills and drugs are prolific. Pills are seen in our society as quick and easy solutions to a broad spectrum of ailments, some of which have nothing to do with medical issues. Doctors have complained for years that patients want nothing more than to walk out of their offices happily holding a prescription. Certainly, swallowing medication is much easier than finding a solution to their problem, such as changing their economic, social, or interpersonal difficulties. Should society expect more from athletes, who might take a pill with hopes of improving their performance rather than the alternative requiring a lot of work and sacrifice?

DISCUSSION QUESTIONS

1. What regulatory body should oversee the use of performance-enhancing drugs?
2. Is it possible that drugs should be allowed in sports? Or even one particular sport?
3. What are the motivations of young athletes to engage in doping?
4. At the university level, what is the NCAA doing about tightening regulations against PEDs?
5. Is drug use a moral issue or merely an ethical issue having to do with fairness?
6. Are there certain types of people/athletes that use PEDs more than others?

REFERENCES

Canseco, J. (2005). *Juiced: Wild times, rampant 'roids, smash hits and how baseball got big.* Regan Books.

Chirico, A., Lucidi, F., Pica, G., Di Santo, D., Galli, F., Alivernini, F., Mallia, L., Zelli, A., Kruglanski, A. W., & Pierro, A. (2021). The motivational underpinnings of intentions to use doping in sport: A sample of young non-professional athletes. *International Journal of Environmental Research and Public Health, 18*(10). https://doi.org/10.3390/ijerph18105411

Murray, T. H. (2018). "Natural" talents and dedication—meanings and values in sport. *American Journal of Bioethics, 18*(6), 1–3. https://doi.org/10.1080/15265161.2018.1474014

Rosen, D. M. (2008). *Dope: A history of performance enhancement in sports from the nineteenth century to today.* Praeger.

Sánchez-Oliver, A. J., Grimaldi-Puyana, M., & Domínguez, R. (2019). Evaluation and behavior of Spanish bodybuilders: Doping and sports supplements. *Biomolecules, 9*(4), 122. https://doi.org/10.3390/biom9040122

Silverberg, S. M. (2010). Safe at home? Assessing U.S. efforts to protect youths from the effects of performance enhancing drugs in sports. *Brooklyn Journal of International Law, 35*(1), 271–310.

Weber, W. S. (2014). Preserving baseball's integrity through proper drug testing: Time for the Major League Baseball Players Association to let go of its collective bargaining reins. *University of Colorado Law Review, 85*(1), 267–312.

Sports, Athletes, Substance Misuse

A Major Gap in Social Work Education

INTRODUCTION

If social work's fundamental mission is to enhance the well-being of all people and pursue economic and social justice (Moya et al., 2018), it would appear that social work practitioners should focus on collegiate athletes and their struggles with mental health and substance use disorders. Gill (2008; 2014; 2017) has continuously called the social work profession and social workers to "enter the game" and participate at the greatest levels possible. Gill and colleagues present a convincing argument for the need to focus on athletes as a vulnerable population in need of social services similar to other vulnerable populations. They present a historical background of social work in sport, beginning with Jane Addams as she served as a de facto athletic director at Hull House when sport activities were embedded within social services for immigrants at Hull House in the 1900s (Gill et al., 2017). From the 1900s to the establishment of the National Alliance of Social Workers in Sports organization in 2015, there has been very limited discussion about social workers helping those in sports. The college social work curricula do not purposely include athletes as one of the vulnerable populations discussed in the classroom. If there is classroom discussion, the focus is on a current news item regarding a specific athlete who may either have criminal charges pending or a team suspension due to substance misuse/abuse. The only reason for the class discussion is typically because the athlete in question is an elite athlete. Thus, from the 1900s to 2015 (establishment of NASWS), there has seldom the link between social workers and athletics in either the literature or social work curricula. This appears to be a grave injustice, especially in light of the fact that the social work profession's mission, according to the Code of Ethics, is to assist vulnerable populations (NASW, 2015) and to provide social and economic justice while remaining current with societal change (CSWE, 2021).

Grobman (2017) describes social work and sport as an emerging specialization with a growing need for social workers to provide services to athletes. He suggests the mission of the NASWS as a reasonable mechanism for strong advocacy for the inclusion of focus on athletes in curricula of the 531 accredited undergraduate social work programs and the 272 accredited graduate social work programs in the United States (CSWE, 2019).

The NASWS focus is on "advocacy for the health and well-being of athletes" (Moore as cited by Grobman, 2017, para. 2). In addition, there is a need for ongoing training and workshops to educate social work professionals on effective therapeutic models (micro level) and strategies that can be utilized when working in partnership with this population on a macro level of practice (team and

TABLE 12.1 2019 Annual Survey Response Rate by Survey Section

	Invitations	Completed Responses	% Responding
Baccalaureate	531	469	88.3
Master's	272	236	86.8
Practice Doctoral (DSW)	18	14	77.8
Research Doctoral (PhD)	80	67	83.8

Source: CSWE 2019 Summary of Annual Survey of Social Work Programs. https://www.cswe.org/CSWE/media/CSWEAnnualReports/CSWE_Annual-Report_19-20.pdf.

community interventions) (ASWIS, n.d.). Although the NASWS is a fairly new organization (established 7 years ago) with only about 50 members, their mission is inclusive of advocating, educating, training, collaborating, and encouraging research in this specialty area (ASWIS, n.d.).

The purpose of this chapter is to continue advocating for the social work profession (CSWE and NASW) and social workers to again stand on the shoulders of Jane Addams and work with athletes, and to encourage and join the members of the NASWS in their quest to include athletes in the study of vulnerable populations in the course curriculum and promote research that will provide and increase attention to the needs of collegiate athletes. Too often, it is forgotten that athletes are humans who also seek fulfillment of basic needs that are essential to the actualization of their goals. The amount of stress and pressures experienced can cause them to become unintentionally self-destructive. They must function as an athlete, as a student, and as a member of the communities (college and home). The expectations are greatest in their role as athlete because there are gains (economic and social) for their performance. Thus, as an athlete, they are tossed into a culture of doing whatever it takes.

DOING WHATEVER IT TAKES

Some athletes may think, "I'll do whatever it takes to win games." Collegiate athletes often use professional athletes as their role models, and the thinking that winning should be the primary focus in sports is highlighted in professional sports. This implies that the athlete must neglect their personal injuries and anything going on in their personal lives to focus on winning and that they are not conscious or aware of the immediate and long-term occupational safety and health risks (OSH) (Chen et al., 2019). There is limited research on OSH. Athletes perform with little awareness about the long-term consequences for playing the sport. The sport culture encourages the continued idea of playing to win the game. If players are injured and leave the game, they are ostracized not only by fans, but by teammates and some coaches for not continuing the play even while injured. This places competitive sports culture in direct conflict with providing safe working conditions (Chen et al., 2019) because "doing whatever it takes" can put many athletes in danger of suffering from mental health and substance use disorders.

Awareness of prevention measures are seldom discussed in collegiate sport. It would be effective to begin the discussions about preventing occupational risks with younger children who participate in sports because the sport culture begins with children's participation at a young age. Although Felfe et al. (2016)

suggest the importance of children participating in sports as a positive enhancer for improving social skills, building team comradery, and improving grades, their research does not extend to the discussion of long-term effects that may impact athletes' lives as they adopt the collegiate and professional sport culture perspective of performing well regardless of the health consequences. Social workers have historically assisted children and their families with biopsychosocial therapeutic approaches. However, not enough focus has been placed on sport culture as a negative influence in child growth and development. As an emerging specialty field of social work practice, it is important to begin to consider how the sport culture impacts attitudes and behaviors so that counseling can be an effective intervention tool for athletes, often dually diagnosed, who are experiencing mental health and substance misuse crises.

Historical Thoughts Between Disciplines

The major gap in social work education has been insensitivity to athletes as a vulnerable population and the reality that many social workers may feel uncomfortable working with dually diagnosed clients. Miller (1999) provides an important descriptive analogy for this discomfort suggesting historical struggles with mental health workers indicating that mental health workers "have not always liked working with alcoholics and addicts" citing the fact that they "lacked knowledge (technique) about how to best treat them" (p. 1). Historically, mental health counselors (social workers) and addiction counselors were separate careers. These counselors knew little about the other's area of specialty, even though many mental disorders are related to alcohol and drug use disorders (Kessler, 2004). Prior to the 1990s mental health issues and addictions were treated separately, and the approach was to treat the addiction first, with the mental illness issue as secondary (ORC, 2021). This combination of mental disorders and alcohol and drug addiction is termed dual diagnosis. Dual diagnosis is often thought to be associated with mental disorders because clients with mental disorders may self-medicate, which can lead to substance or drug misuse and addiction. However, the reverse can also occur with the client who experiments with illegal or prescription drugs for a period of time and develops a mental disorder as a result of continued drug misuse/abuse. The discussion becomes which came first—the addiction or the mental illness?

This question is answered with each individual client, but both must be treated. Even though the client may identify one disorder and not the other, the social worker must explore and probe to ensure that both disorders are treated. The thinking that if the mental disorder is treated the addiction will simply go away is separation of the disorders primarily because the counselor has not been trained to address both disorders. Although CSWE convened a group in 2019 to design and implement the inclusion of substance misuse/abuse into the curricula of accredited social work programs, there is still no mention of applying these newfound curricula to athletes.

Social workers are now obtaining training in addictions to address the issues related to dual diagnosis. However, this implies the need to become dually licensed (licensed social worker and licensed addiction specialist). If the counselor does not possess both licensures, the counselor will be practicing outside of their scope of practice. *Comorbidity* is often a concept utilized interchangeably with the concept of *dual diagnosis*. However, comorbidity is a broader concept with the application extended to any illness, such as hypertension and depression, and these disorders do not have to be concurrent (Magobet, 2020) but can occur concurrently and unrelated to another medical issue (Lesser, 2021). Thus, when clients are dually diagnosed, the counselor has to "untangle" the overlapping symptoms that may be presenting.

Miller (1999) states that historically mental health workers were not sure how to work with addicted clients because these clients experienced a "different" pattern of behavior during the treatment process with lying, relapsing, and being noncompliant with authority figures (p. 26). This suggests that mental health workers viewed themselves as "professional" and addiction counselors as primarily individual grassroots peer counselors who had experienced addiction and the cycle of addiction. This historical distancing between the two disciplines made it difficult for clients to receive holistic treatment without referral. However, with the pharmaceutical price frenzy, the Medicare surge, establishment of the National Alliance on Mental Illness (NAMI), and the need to centralize treatment, the two disciplines have seemingly formed a collaborative effort to formulate treatment for dually diagnosed clients. The development of the concept of dual diagnosis in the late 1980s created mandated treatment services, clarification of treatment service concerns, and development of the integrative approaches to working with mental health and substance abusing clients (Drake & Wallach, 2000). It was only in 1998 that the Substance Abuse and Mental Health Services Administration (SAMHSA), along with Center for Substance Abuse Treatment (CSAT), developed the competencies for addiction counselors. The Technical Assistance Publication Series (TAP) provides information on effective clinical counseling for clients with substance use disorders. It includes the knowledge, skills, and attitudes that counselors should demonstrate to master each of the competency areas (SAMHSA, 1998; 2017).

What If You Want to Counsel Athletes?

Those who want to counsel athletes need at least a bachelor's degree in counseling. Knowledge and skills in addictions is strongly encouraged, and licensure in addiction is recommended. Many athletes struggle with the pressures of the sport and too many that are encouraged to win may use PEDs to recover from injury faster and get back into the game. Or some may unintentionally become addicted to alcohol and other illegal drugs. The NCAA national survey reported that 22.3% of college students reported recently using illicit drugs while use among athletes is greater (as cited by the American Addiction Centers, 2021). These athletes are not receiving therapeutic assistance, and there is a need to increase the number of licensed addiction counselors in America because clinical therapeutic intervention with athletes should make the starting lineup (BLS, 2021).

Substance abuse counselors provide the needed treatment for clients who are struggling with alcoholism and other addictions. States require counselors to be licensed by a state board in order to practice. Educational requirements differ from state to state. If private clinical practice is a goal, clinical experience may be a requirement (3,000 hours). In some graduate school programs, the substance abuse certificate is an option as an area of specialty. After the applicant has obtained the necessary requirements for certification, an application to the state board may be necessary to add the substance abuse specialty.

Based on the Bureau of Labor Statistics (BLS, 2021), substance abuse counselors are employed with a mean annual wage of $53,550 (with 2 years of experience). This area of specialty is projected to increase in demand. Some states, such as North Carolina, are aggressively recruiting substance counselors with scholarship stipends and other incentives such as payment for supervision, testing, and applications to encourage or ensure that the specialty area will increase the pool of competent substance practitioners.

Many athletes, by the nature of their roles, may be experiencing mental illness and substance misuse or substance use disorders. They may be depressed about an injury that has caused them to delay their

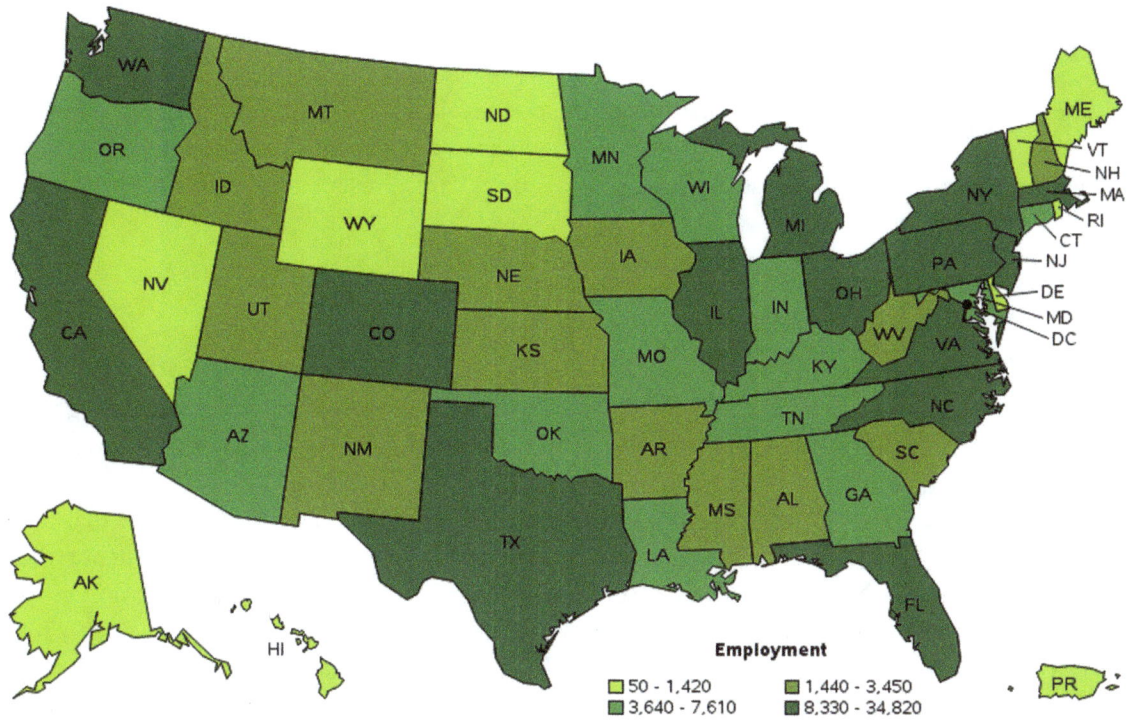

FIGURE 12.1 *Employment of Substance Abuse, Behavioral Disorder, and Mental Health Counselors by State, May 2020*

game time and decide to double their PEDs to quickly get back into the game. Although their intent is to win games, the consequences can become lethal. When working with dually diagnosed clients such as athletes, the counseling process may take longer due to the dual aspects of the client's condition, which may be cause for multidimensional approaches. In addition, few clinical practitioners are qualified to work with the dually diagnosed client. Social workers do not understand the need to be competent to work with this population. Competencies must be included within social work practice skills in academic institutions of higher learning to encourage the dual licensure by social workers (both LCAS and LCSW licensures) and include addiction as one of the required CEUs for renewal of the LCSW licensure. Addiction training should be required for clinical supervisors, along with CEUs.

When counseling athletes, it is critical to remember that one size does not fit all. Although athletes publicly display a team comradery, many are lonely individuals experiencing a roller coaster ride without ability to receive assistance to move off the roller coaster. An athlete may display mental confusion, detachment, strained personal relationships, feelings of uncertainty, and anger. As a means of coping, many may isolate themselves for fear that their vulnerabilities will be displayed and discovered. Many may self-medicate to ease their pain (e.g., emotional as well as physical). Some even become involved in risky behavior, such as large consumption of alcohol and other drugs. An essential factor to remember when counseling athletes is to focus on all the issues causing the client discomfort and to establish goals and objectives with the client to address each of the identified areas. There are different levels of treatment, and the severity of the identified problem can determine the level of treatment.

LEVELS OF TREATMENT

Level of care is the type of treatment that an athlete may need, based on the counselor's assessment of the condition. The assessment process takes place when the counselor begins the exploratory activity with the client in the form of questions based on historical and present information. Questions may include the following:

- At what age did you begin to use _____?
- How often did you use _____?
- How much _____ do you use?

These questions along with others will allow the counselor to make some deduction regarding the level of care (treatment) needed. The different levels of addiction rehabilitation treatment are categorized as inpatient, outpatient, and detoxification.

Detoxification involves removing toxic matter from the body to stabilize the client so that physical symptoms of dependency (withdrawal) can be managed with less harm to the client. Inpatient treatment can be considered the least intrusive and more personable. Some examples of detoxification programs according to National Center for Complementary and Integrative Health (NCCIH, 2019) include fasting, drinking only juices, eating certain foods, taking dietary supplements, and using homeopathy herbs. Even though detox is widely used, the research is sparse and conflicting on the effects of detoxification. Medical detoxification involves the 24/7 monitoring by a nurse with a physician on call if needed. Residential inpatient (such as hospitalization) involves the client remaining within a treatment facility to obtain necessary intense monitoring from professional staff. While inpatient care provides residential care and comfort for clients, outpatient care allows the client to remain in the home while attending treatment programs in the community under the supervision of the referring counselor, a nurse practitioner, or a medical doctor. Inpatient care is typically provided in a hospital or facility until the physician discharges the patient (in a group home the counselor's signature would be needed in order to terminate the client). ASAM criteria is generally utilized for these levels of care.

ASAM criteria are used in many treatment facilities focused on substance addiction. In 1991, The National Association of Addiction Treatment Providers and The American Society of Addiction Medicine created the ASAM standardized patient placement criteria (Chuang et al., 2009), which is used throughout the country.

The Assessment Process

The assessment should not become an oversimplified process. It is important to consider all aspects of issues presented by the athlete. Therefore, the counselor should begin the process with allowing the athlete to identify the problem(s). The search for the nature and cause of the problem is essential, explored with the client by probing for information that will assist with understanding the problem. Historical information regarding type of substance used, frequency, dose, and effects should be explored with the client. In addition, it is critical to understand the athlete's culture and cultural norms to guard against decisions that may hinder or limit successful treatment outcomes.

A cursory lens of an assessment interview when recording the clinical notes can consist of identification of the problem (from athlete's perspective as well as what the counselor hears and observes), factual information collected (information from the referral case file), list of unanswered questions for further probing (any inconsistencies between the athlete's lens and information obtained from the case file), and recommendations (during the early phrase of the counseling process the recommendation may be continued sessions containing assessment measurement tools such as the MAST or ASI to provide further information regarding the athlete's situation). Some useful measurement tools have been discussed in chapter 10. The DSM-5 should be used to make the diagnosis. It is critical to remember that the diagnosis provides the foundation for the treatment plan. The treatment plan includes the athlete's goals (short-term and long-term) and objectives, roles and responsibilities, activities, and time frames for meeting the goals and objectives. The athlete's compliance in the treatment process and the level of care will determine the prioritization of the goals and objectives. In addiction counseling, the including significant others as support is a very useful aspect of the treatment process.

One major challenge to the treatment process for collegiate athletes may be the coach or trainers. Therefore, it is important for the counselor to overcome this barrier with initial discussions with the athlete during the signing of the confidentiality and release of information forms. The coach can play a significant role in a successful outcome if the coach is a support of the counseling process. Often coaches with athletes in therapy want to know if the athlete can continue to play the sport and how long the treatment process will take. Coaches should not be included in the treatment process if they cannot honor the privacy and confidentiality of the athlete in accordance with the federal regulations (42 C.F.R., Part 2).

Treatment plans should be clear and comprehensive. Some agencies will have treatment forms, but clinical practitioners in private practice may struggle with developing treatment plans. An example of a treatment plan format follows.

TREATMENT PLAN

Referral source: _____ Referral date _____

Client's name _____ DOB _____ Race _____ Gender _____

Date entered treatment _____

Diagnosis: _____

Brief history:

| Short-term goals | Intervention | Time frame | Measurement tool |

| Long-term goals | Intervention | Time frame | Measurement tool |

Clinical Impressions

Next scheduled appointment date/time

Client's signature _____   Date _____

Counselor's signature _____   Date _____

PROVIDE AN ASSESSMENT AND TREATMENT PLAN FOR JOHN DOE

John Doe is a 22-year-old freshman attending a major university in America. He was spotted and sought by recruiters from more than 10 different colleges and universities since he was a sophomore in high school football. He is from a small rural town in Mississippi. His family consists of mother as head of the household and six younger siblings. The family had struggled financially as John Doe's mother became ill and unable to work. As a freshman in high school, John Doe worked in the country store, devoting little time to studies or social activities. But his enjoyment of football was recognized by many recruiters and coaches as he took his team to the national championship (which had never occurred in the history of his high school). His ability to pass the football to players and out maneuver tackles was astounding to everyone.

His first year at the university he selected to attend has been an exciting whirlwind for him and his family. John Doe continued his unbelievable performances in his freshman year at the top 10 university, taking the team to defeat Notre Dame, Michigan State, and Ohio State. Then John Doe's mother died of heart disease, and his sibling were placed in foster care. No one discussed this with John Doe because the coach simply stated that he would take care of John Doe and not to worry about anything. Teammates attempted to "cheer" John Doe with drinking parties. He continued to drink even when there were no parties. Becoming fearful that he would be released from the team, he drank alcohol daily. In practice, John Doe was on the field without appropriate gear, took a hit from a teammate, and did not get up. After release from the hospital, John Doe was told by doctors that he was "lucky" that he only fractured his arm. "It could have been your throwing shoulder," said one medical professional. He was given oxycodone to relieve the pain. John continued to drink, and when he felt pain, he would also take a pill. His prescription was renewed without question, and he continued this pattern. But his game performance diminished, and he was replaced with a backup. His coach and teammates spent less time with him, and he was not sure what was happening. John Doe phoned his grocery store boss who was in retirement and indicated that he had no one and did not know what to do. In the little town of Horseshoe, Mississippi, there was one social worker, and the grocery store boss asked her to call John Doe.

You are the social worker. How would you assist John Doe?
Hint: Provide an assessment
Develop a treatment plan

GAPS IN ADDICTION COUNSELING

There is a gap in continued education for incorporating treatment and assessment measures in clinical practice (Wilson & Johnson, 2013) and for counselors who are working in both the addiction and social work disciplines. Just as social work education is not prepared for change, addiction counselors are in a similar state of anomie. This developing area of specialty (clinical addiction counseling) is not without the need for continued education, training, and treatment strategies derived from the understanding about the nature of addiction problems (Thombs & Osborn, 2001). There is still the overall prevailing notion that the disease model is the dominate model of practice. Although this model has its merits and has served the purpose of making attempts at unifying addiction thinking, there is need for more research to provide current data on not only the disease model of practice, but to introduce and encourage other models for consideration. Many treatment programs have typically selected approaches based on personal recovery experiences (Thombs & Osborn, 2001).

It is time for change (Thombs & Osborn, 2001). One size should not fit all clients. The disease model provided its usefulness at a time when little was known about addictions other than the moral attribute that individuals knew right from wrong and could stop using at any given moment. However, there is a desperate need to expose graduate social work students to other lenses that prove useful in the treatment process. Social work students should be introduced to not only the moral and disease models but also psychodynamic, social learning, sociocultural, and public health models.

The harm reduction model is also a consideration when the client is not at the point of addiction. It is an alternative approach to the abstinence model and continues to be the subject of extensive debate. The goal of the harm reduction model is to assist clients to avoid harm (O'Hare, 2007) to themselves and society without morally judging the client. Harm reduction is based on three considerations: (1) there is a continuum of risky behaviors that range from minimum to extreme, (2) any change or movement in the direction of reducing harm is positive, and (3) sobriety is not for everyone (Guthmann et al., 2000).

Although groups and group work are essential curriculum components in accredited social work programs, the discussions are seldom focused on working with substance abusing clients. SAMHSA (2015) supports group models and identifies the following five common models used in substance abuse treatment:

- psychoeducational (clients focus on substance abuse education);
- skills development groups (identify and strengthen skills that will assist with reduction and elimination of risky behaviors leading to abuse);
- cognitive-behavioral groups (changing the thoughts that lead to abuse);
- support groups (provide a forum for sharing information and obtaining support); and
- interpersonal process groups (developmental issues that contribute to abuse and relapse).

Social work and addiction counseling have grown substantially and continue to evolve, establishing their individual entities within the disciplines. Historically the evolution has not been without its debates as social workers advocated for the professionalization of addiction counselors and their roles and addiction counselors advocated for transitioning from a moralistic model to a disease model of consideration. Although the label "mental health and substance abuse counseling" implies a separation, there is some overlap in the delivery of services. Both can provide mental health services. The role of the social worker is broader, but they should not practice outside their scope of practice, which is defined by each state legally based on the ethical standards as delineated by each of the disciplines.

SUMMARY

Although social workers are playmakers (Newman et al., 2021) and have been working with adolescents who may have been engaged in sports activities, the focus has not been on social work and sport. Some social work programs may discuss athletes and sport; however, there is no clear delineation of the role/

responsibility of the social worker, nor are there comprehensive strategies to assist clinical practitioners when counseling athletes. Athletes are not viewed in social work programs as vulnerable. The emerging attention has erupted due to effort and advocation by the NASWS organization. This organization provides reasonable discussion and explanations for the call for NASW and CSWE to strongly consider including sports as a field of specialty in the social work discipline. Athletes are not considered a vulnerable population because of the fame and fortune that comes with the sport. However, the price of their fame and fortune is seldom realized. Many athletes suffer in silence with the pressures from coaches, trainers, families, fans, and academics. They live in an isolated yet turbulent environment of the collegiate athletic department on campuses of higher education. They are stigmatized if they seek therapeutic assistance and cut from the team with a loss of scholarship if they do not seek assistance and sink into a state of depression, which can spiral to further vulnerability and suicide ideation.

The mission of social work is to provide assistance, especially to vulnerable populations, and to ensure social justice. Social workers should become the change agent for collegiate athletes and those young aspiring athletes in middle and high school who are increasingly using PEDs and illegal drugs as they seek to do whatever it takes to perform well for their coaches and team. Social workers have the values, knowledge, and skills to provide athletic counseling, not only to athletes but to coaches as well. Just as the importance of social workers is emerging within physician's offices, these professionals should become critical resources within the athletic departments in higher education.

In addition to inclusion of sports in social work, this chapter encourages more research in sport settings. Social work is the most reasonable discipline to assist with the well-being of athletes, and it is likely that more collegiate athletes can accomplish academic success while succeeding in their sport. Thus, social workers must begin to enter sports games. A major challenge for social workers is feeling ill prepared to work with this population, primarily due to limited exposure in social work curricula. Training must integrate approaches to treatment for dually diagnosed clients, along with the willingness to rethink the concept of vulnerable populations to include athletes as an underserved group.

DISCUSSION QUESTIONS

1. On the internet, select your state to determine the state requirements to become a licensed addiction counselor: https://sobercollege.com/substance-use-counselor/counseling-requirements-state/

   Discuss your findings in a group.

2. Identify some challenges to bridging the gap between social work and sport. Discuss with a group strategies for overcoming the challenges.
3. What is your understanding of the disease model of addictions? How is it similar to the harm reduction model, and how is it different?
4. In a group, discuss what is meant by dual diagnosis and provide examples. What are your thoughts regarding the thinking that athletes are a vulnerable population?
5. What are your thoughts about the idea that many social workers are ill prepared to provide treatment to athletes? What should occur in order to bring about change?

REFERENCES

Alliance of Social Workers in Sports (ASWIS). (n.d.). About Alliance of Social Workers in Sports. https://www.aswis.org/about

American Addiction Centers (AAC). (2021). College athletes and substance use: A look at drug use by gender and sport. https://www.projectknow.com/discover/college-athletes-and-substance-use/

Bureau of Labor Statistics (BLS). (2021). Occupational employment and wages, May 2021, 21-1018 Substance Abuse, Behavioral Disorder, and Mental Health Counselors. https://www.bls.gov/oes/current/oes211018.htm

Chuang, E., Wells, R., Alexander, J. A., Friedmann, P. D., & Lee, I. H. (2009). Factors associated with use of ASAM criteria and service provision in a national sample of outpatient substance abuse treatment units. *Journal of Addiction Medicine, 3*(3), 139–150. https://doi.org/10.1097/ADM.0b013e31818ebb6f; https://www.ncbi.nlm.nih.gov/pmc/articles/PMC3584172/

CSWE. (2019). *Statistics on social work education in the U.S. Summary of CSWE annual survey of social work programs.* https://cswe.org/getattachment/Research-Statistics/2019-Annual-Statistics-on-Social-Work-Education-in-the-United-States-Final-(1).pdf.aspx

CSWE. (2021). Social, economic, and environmental justice. https://www.cswe.org/events-meetings/2021-apm/proposals/2021-apm-tracks/social,-economic,-and-environmental-justice/

Drake, R. E., & Wallach, M. A. (2000). Dual diagnosis: 15 years of progress. *Psychiatric Services, 51*(9), 1126–1129. https://doi.org/10.1176/appi.ps.51.9.1126; https://ps.psychiatryonline.org/doi/full/10.1176/appi.ps.51.9.1126

Felfe, C., Lechner, M., & Steinmayr, A. (2016). Sports and child development. *PLoS ONE 11*(5), e0151729. https://journals.plos.org/plosone/article?id=10.1371/journal.pone.0151729

Gill, E. L., Jr. (2008). Mental health in college athletics: It's time for social work to get in the game. *Social Work, 53*(1), 85–88. https://www.jstor.org/stable/23721192

Gill, E. L., Jr. (2014). Integrating collegiate sports into social work education. *Journal of Social Work Education, 50*(2), 305–321. doi: 10.1080/10437797.2014.856245; https://www.tandfonline.com/doi/abs/10.1080/10437797.2014.856245

Gill, E. L., Rowan, D., & Moore, M. (2017). Special issue editors' note: The role of social work practice, advocacy, and research in college athletics. *Journal of Issues in Intercollegiate Athletics*, 1–10. http://csri-jiia.org/wp-content/uploads/2017/07/JIIA_2017_SI_00.pdf

Grobman, A. (2017). Social work gets in the game. *The New Social Worker.* https://www.socialworker.com/feature-articles/practice/social-work-gets-in-the-game/

Guthmann, D. (with Sandberg, K., & Lybarger, R.). (2000, March 23–24). Models of alcohol and other drug treatment for considerations when working with deaf and hard of hearing individuals. *Proceedings from Stepping Forward: Creative Approaches in Prevention, Treatment and Recovery for Deaf People.* Minneapolis, Minnesota. http://www.mncddeaf.org/articles/models_ad.htm

Kessler, R. C. (2004). The epidemiology of dual diagnosis. *Biological Psychiatry, 56*(10), 730–737. https://www.sciencedirect.com/science/article/abs/pii/S0006322304007395

Lesser, W. B. (2021). Comorbidity testing and evaluations. https://dualdiagnosis.org/testing-assessments-comorbidity/

Li, Y., Chen, P. Y., Tuckey, M. R., McLinton, S. S., & Dollard, M. F. (2019). Prevention through job design: Identifying high-risk job characteristics associated with workplace bullying. *Journal of Occupational Health Psychology, 24*(2), 297–306. https://doi.org/10.1037/ocp0000133

Magobet, V. (2020, January 8). What is the Difference: Comorbidity and dual diagnosis vs. co-occurring disorders. https://diamondhousedetox.com/comorbidity-dual-diagnosis-cooccurring-disorder/

Miller, G. A. (1999). *Learning the language of addiction counseling.* Allyn & Bacon.

Moore, M. A. (2016). Do psychosocial services make the starting lineup? Providing services to student-athletes. *Journal of Animal Science, 2*, 50–74. https://journals.ku.edu/jams/article/view/5046

Moya, E. M., Chavez-Baray, S. M., Martinez, O., Mattera, B., & Adcox, C. (2018). Bridging the gap between micro and macro practice to address homelessness in the U.S.–Mexico border region: Implications for practitioners and community stakeholders. *Reflections (Long Beach, Calif.), 24*(1), 102–118. (nih.gov)

NASW. (2015). NASW Code of Ethics. https://www.socialworkers.org/About/Ethics/Code-of-Ethics/Code-of-Ethics-English

National Center for Complementary and Integrative Health (NCCIH). (2019). "Detoxes" and "cleanses": What you need to know. NIH. U.S. Department of Health and Human Services. https://www.nccih.nih.gov/health/detoxes-and-cleanses-what-you-need-to-know

Newman, T. J., Magier, E., Okamoto, K., Kimiecik, C., Shute, L., Beasley, L., & Tucker, A. R. (2021). Social work in sport: Playmakers in the athletic arena. *Journal of Social Work, 22*(3), 692–714. https://doi.org/10.1177/14680173211009743; https://journals.sagepub.com/doi/abs/10.1177/14680173211009743

O'Hare P. (2007). Merseyside, the first harm reduction conferences, and the early history of harm reduction. *International Journal of Drug Policy, 18*(2), 141–144. https://pubmed.ncbi.nlm.nih.gov/17689357/

ORC. (2021). Dual diagnosis treatment centers of Los Angeles and Malibu California. Oro House Recovery Centers. https://www.ororecovery.com/dual-diagnosis-treatment-centers-in-malibu-california/?gclid=EAIaIQobChMIiKvo_fSl9QIVCYizCh16ZwxkEAAYAyAAEgJ0P_D_BwE

SAMHSA. (1998; 2017). *Addiction counseling competencies: The knowledge, skills, and attitudes of professional practice.* U.S. Department of Health and Human Services. https://store.samhsa.gov/sites/default/files/d7/priv/sma12-4171.pdf

SAMHSA. (2015). Substance abuse treatment: Group therapy. A Treatment Improvement Protocol (TIP 41). U.S. Department of Health and Human Services. https://store.samhsa.gov/sites/default/files/d7/priv/sma15-3991.pdf

Thombs, D. L., & Osborn, C. J. (2001). A cluster analytic study of clinical orientations among chemical dependency counselors. *Journal of Counseling and Development, 79*, 450–458. https://www.semanticscholar.org/paper/A-Cluster-Analytic-Study-of-Clinical-Orientations-Thombs-Osborn/348c8c4d05c5c514d7c8791b1b2520607aef1a0e

Wilson, A. D., & Johnson, P. (2013). Counselors' understanding of process addiction: A blind spot in the counseling field. *The Professional Counselor, 3*, 16–22. https://www.semanticscholar.org/paper/Counselors'-Understanding-of-Process-Addiction%3A-A-Wilson-Johnson/284d57cc911a73897e99ec5f961f066cb2292068

IMAGE CREDIT

Fig. 12.1: Source: https://www.bls.gov/oes/current/oes211018.htm.

Future Challenges in Athletes Who Use Performance-Enhancing Drugs

INTRODUCTION

Athletes rely on a number of strategies to help them remain competitive in their sports. One of these strategies, albeit an illicit one, is the use of performance-enhancing drugs. Up to 4 million Americans have used anabolic-androgenic steroids (AAS), a group of illicit drugs designed to increase muscle mass for the purposes of athletic performance or personal appearance (Baggish et al., 2017). The lifetime prevalence of AAS use in men ranges from 1% to 5%. These drugs are more commonly used by males than females at a ratio of 50 to 1 (Anawalt, 2019, p. 2491). Approximately 1 million individuals, primarily male, become dependent on these drugs, resulting in long-term use (Anawalt, 2019, p. 2491; Baggish et al., 2017).

Anabolic-androgenic steroids are synthetic derivatives of testosterone, which has masculinizing effects. These types of drugs come in several different forms, including oral, injectable, and transdermic gel. They help to increase muscle mass by increasing the production of actin and myosin, key skeletal muscle proteins (La Vignera et al., 2018, p. 3). Substances commonly taken in conjunction with AAS include erythropoietin, growth hormone, insulin-like growth factor, diuretics, thyroid hormone, and opioids for pain (Chang et al., 2018, p. 736). Despite the use of these other substances and their potential effects, the focus of the following discussion is on the long-term effects of AAS. Athletes who use AAS may experience in the future a number of long-term effects that impact cardiovascular health, fertility and reproductive health, psychiatric and cognitive functioning, and several other body functions.

LONG-TERM EFFECTS OF AAS USE

Cardiovascular

Athletes who use AAS may experience long-term negative cardiovascular effects. Baggish et al. (2017) compared the cardiovascular function of 86 former AAS-using weight lifters with 54 nonusing weight lifters. Results indicated that male athletes with a history of AAS use demonstrated higher blood pressure, a higher rate of dyslipidemia, and a higher resting heart rate. In addition, these athletes exhibited a greater left ventricular mass and thicker left ventricular walls. Overall, their left ventricular function, in which oxygen rich blood is pumped by the heart to the rest of the body, was poorer than athletes who did not use these performance-enhancing drugs. Anabolic androgenic steroid users also demonstrated a higher coronary plaque volume and increased atherosclerosis, which could eventually lead to artery blockages and heart attacks (Baggish et al., 2017).

The use of AAS is also associated with heart dysfunction and clotting disorders. According to Chang et al. (2018), AAS may increase the levels of proteins involved in coagulation, thus reducing clotting time (p. 737). In addition, these drugs create an increased risk for thrombosis, and the blood clots formed could lead to blocked arteries (p. 742). Horwitz et al. (2019) reported that previous AAS users demonstrated a five-fold increase in clotting disorders, as well as three-fold increases in cardiomyopathy and atrial fibrillation (p. 336).

Fertility and Reproductive Health

The use of AAS by athletes may negatively impact their future fertility and reproductive health. For example, the use of AAS in conjunction with exogenous testosterone is associated with erectile dysfunction (Sansone et al., 2018, p. 7). In fact, users of AAS reported a three-fold increase in medication used to treat erectile dysfunction when compared with nonusers (Horwitz et al., 2019, p. 336). Males may experience testicular shrinkage and apoptosis, or death, of male germ cells (Sansone et al., 2018, p. 7). Users of these drugs are at a 2.4-fold increased risk for infertility (Horwitz et al., 2019, p. 336). However, low sperm counts and the absence of sperm cells can resolve in less than one year after discontinuation of AAS (Sansone et al., 2018, p. 7). Users may also experience a loss of libido (Bagge et al., 2017, p. 816) and a 13-fold increase in the incidence of gynecomastia, in which males develop excessive breast tissue (Horwitz et al., 2019, p. 335). Other performance-enhancing drugs may also negatively impact reproductive health. Beta blockers, which are used to reduce anxiety and tremors in precision sports, can delay or lead to the complete loss of ejaculation. And diuretics and amphetamines can impair erectile function and fertility (Sansone et al., 2018, p. 8).

Males are not the only athletes that can be affected by performance-enhancing drugs. According to La Vignera et al. (2018), AAS use in women can lead to an enlarged clitoris and changes to menstruation, including the complete loss of menstruation and ovulation. Women may also experience breast atrophy and the development of male characteristics such as male pattern baldness, excessive hair growth, and a lowering of the voice due to the thickening of vocal cords (p. 4). Postmenopausal women with a history of AAS use demonstrate an increased risk of breast cancer (p. 5). However, it is important to note that although an association between breast cancer and AAS use exists in this population, there is no causal evidence. It is also important to note that there is a lack of well-documented studies regarding the reversibility of the effects with cessation of drug use (p. 5).

Psychiatric and Cognitive

In addition to impacting the heart and the reproductive systems, AAS use can negatively impact the brain. Bagge et al. (2017) surveyed 996 former elite male athletes regarding past AAS use and health problems. This sample had a mean age of 57 years, and 21% of the athletes were former AAS users. Individuals who used these drugs were more likely to experience depression and anxiety than nonusers. In addition, advanced users, or those who used AAS for more than 2 years, were more likely than more unaccustomed users to experience depression, psychosis, and anxiety (p. 816).

Hauger et al. (2019) also reported on the cognitive and psychiatric effects of AAS use. The purpose of this mixed methods study was to compare AAS users with and without dependence on the drugs and nonusers with respect to their ability to recognize emotions in others. Researchers used semi-structured interviews to gather data regarding the history and nature of drug use in participants. In addition, the researchers used the Structured Clinical Interview for DSM-IV Axis II Personality Disorders (SCID II) to assess for drug dependence and urinalysis to assess for current drug use. Participants completed an emotion biological motion task in which they viewed video clips of people expressing emotions through body language rather than facial expression. Participants were then asked to identify the type of emotion expressed in each video clip (p. 2669). Results indicated that a number of differences existed between dependent and nondependent AAS users and those who never used the drugs. For example, nonusers demonstrated the highest IQ, followed by nondependent users and dependent users. Dependent users scored the highest on the SCID II depression scale and the scales for anxiety, ADHD, and antisocial behaviors. These results do not necessarily imply causation, but rather demonstrate an association between AAS use and these negative outcomes (p. 2670). Overall, dependent users demonstrated a reduced ability to recognize emotions, particularly fear, when compared with nondependent users and nonusers (p. 2671). The authors concluded that dependence on AAS could lead to more interpersonal problems and antisocial behavior in the future (p. 2674).

It is possible that these cognitive and psychiatric effects of AAS use are due in part to drug-related physiological changes in the brain. Bjornebekk et al. (2017) compared magnetic resonance images of the brains of male weight lifters who used AAS with images of those who did not use in order to identify any differences in brain structure. Results from the imaging indicated that AAS users possessed a smaller cortical volume and a thinner cortex. These effects increased with longer use of the drugs. These findings are important because the cortex is responsible for higher order brain functions, such as memory, thoughts, and perception (p. 299). The authors concluded that heavy AAS use may be associated with deterioration of brain tissue. This deterioration may be caused by drug-induced death of neurons, although the exact mechanism by which this cell death occurs remains unclear (p. 300).

Other Effects

Several other long-term effects of AAS use are noted in the literature. For example, drug users are more likely to experience tendon rupture, particularly those who have used the drugs for longer than 2 years (Bagge et al., 2017, p. 816). These individuals may also have a higher risk of gallbladder disease (Bagge et al., 2017, p. 816) and a two-fold increase in the incidence of acne (Horwitz et al., 2019, p. 336). With respect to overall mortality rates, users of AAS demonstrate a three-fold increase in mortality when compared to athletes who have never used the drugs (Horwitz et al., 2019, p. 335).

SUMMARY

While the majority of male and female athletes may not use performance-enhancing drugs such as AAS, those who do may face health problems in the future. The use of AAS is associated with negative cardiovascular effects such as poor heart function and an increased risk for clotting. Both males and females who take these drugs may experience problems with fertility and reproductive health. For example, males may develop erectile dysfunction, infertility, or excessive breast tissue. Females may lose breast tissue, develop male characteristics, and experience changes to menstruation and ovulation, the latter of which can affect fertility. Other physical effects may include tendon ruptures, gallbladder disease, acne, and increased risk of mortality. The effects persist beyond the physical. Changes in brain structure associated with AAS use can lead to psychiatric and cognitive deficits, such as a lower IQ or an increased risk of anxiety and depression.

It is important to note that while the literature provides evidence of a link between these effects and AAS use, it does not provide causal evidence. In other words, the studies summarized in this discussion do not directly attribute AAS use to the effects observed. Instead, statistically significant associations were noted. It is always possible that other confounding factors or variables may contribute to the outcomes reported. Overall, however, the evidence overwhelmingly supports the idea that use of AAS among athletes to enhance their performance may lead to a future filled with physical and psychological health problems. Thus, it is important to educate athletes about the long-term effects of AAS use and to create policies that make it more difficult for athletes to obtain these drugs.

DISCUSSION QUESTIONS

1. Aside from the physical and psychological effects associated with AAS use, what moral or ethical issues exist with the use of these drugs by athletes?
2. Should the manufacturers of AAS and other performance-enhancing drugs be held liable for the negative long-term effects? Why or why not?
3. Should athletes who take medications that may be considered "performance enhancing" to treat valid medical conditions be exempt from policies that prohibit the use of these drugs? Why or why not?

REFERENCES

Anawalt, B. D. (2019). Diagnosis and management of anabolic androgenic steroid use. *The Journal of Clinical Endocrinology & Metabolism, 104*(7), 2490–2500. doi: 10.1210/jc.2018-01882

Bagge, A. S. L., Rosén, T., Fahlke, C., Ehrnborg, C., Eriksson, B. O., Moberg, T., & Thiblin, I. (2017). Somatic effects of AAS abuse: A 30-years follow-up study of male former power sports athletes. *Journal of Science and Medicine in Sport, 20*(9), 814–818. http://dx.doi.org/10.1016/j.jsams.2017.03.008

Baggish, A. L., Weiner, R. B., Kanayama, G., Hudson, J. I., Lu, M. T., Hoffmann, U., & Pope, H. G., Jr. (2017). Cardiovascular toxicity of illicit anabolic-androgenic steroid use. *Circulation, 135*(21). https://www.ncbi.nlm.nih.gov/pmc/articles/PMC5614517/

Bjørnebekk, A., Walhovd, K. B., Jørstad, M. L., Due-Tønnessen, P., Hullstein, I. R., & Fjell, A. M. (2017). Structural brain imaging of long-term anabolic-androgenic steroid users and nonusing weightlifters. *Biological Psychiatry, 82*(4), 294–302. doi: 10.1016/j.biopsych.2016.06.017

Chang, S., Münster, A. M. B., Gram, J., & Sidelmann, J. J. (2018). Anabolic androgenic steroid abuse: The effects on thrombosis risk, coagulation, and fibrinolysis. *Seminars in Thrombosis and Hemostasis, 44*(8), 734–746. doi:10.1055/s-0038-1670639

Hauger, L. E., Sagoe, D., Vaskinn, A., Arnevik, E. A., Leknes, S., Jørstad, M. L., & Bjørnebekk, A. (2019). Anabolic androgenic steroid dependence is associated with impaired emotion recognition. *Psychopharmacology, 236*(9), 2667–2676. https://doi.org/10.1007/s00213-019-05239-7

Horwitz, H., Andersen, J. T., & Dalhoff, K. P. (2019). Health consequences of androgenic anabolic steroid use. *Journal of Internal Medicine, 285*(3), 333–340. doi: 10.1111/joim.12850

La Vignera, S., Condorelli, R. A., Cannarella, R., Duca, Y., & Calogero, A. E. (2018). Sport, doping and female fertility. *Reproductive Biology and Endocrinology, 16*(1), 1–10. https://doi.org/10.1186/s12958-018-0437-8

Sansone, A., Sansone, M., Vaamonde, D., Sgrò, P., Salzano, C., Romanelli, F., Lenzi, A., & Di Luigi, L. (2018). Sport, doping and male fertility. *Reproductive Biology and Endocrinology, 16*(114), 1–12. https://doi.org/10.1186/s12958-018-0435-x

INDEX

A
academic integrity, 105–106
academics, 60
acceptance, 6, 25, 45
Adair, C., 66
Addams, J., 125
addiction counseling, 132–133
addiction treatment, 83–86. *See also* treatment
affirmations, 42
African Americans in sports, 52
American Society of Addiction Medicine (ASAM), 88
anabolic-androgenic steroids (AAS), 137–139
anger, 15, 45
anti-anxiety medications, 87
anxiety and depression, 96
assessment in treatment, 84
assessment process, 130–132
athlete(s), 57–69. *See also* college athletes; professional athletes
  academics and, 60
  challenges of trans athletes, 62–65
  continued competitiveness, 61–62
  counseling for, 98–99
  mental game challenges, 57–58
  mental health, 61–62
  physical challenges, 58–59
  physical health, 61–62
  prevalence of drug use among, 5–6
  professional, 6
  social activities and, 60–61
  substance abuse in, 1–2
  success or lack of success, 61
  technological challenges in sports industry, 65–69
athlete behavior, 27–46
  biological theories, 34–36
  critical theories, 36–39
  need to study theory, 28–29
  psychological theories, 30–34
  sociological theories, 29–30
  therapeutic interventions, 39–45

B
Bagge, A. S. L., 138
Baggish, A. L., 137
Bandura, A., 30
bargaining, 45
Beck, A. T., 41
behavior. *See* athlete behavior
Bell, D., 38
Biden, J., 63
Biles, S., 58
biological theories, 34–36
Blackwell, H. B., 37
Blumer, H., 29
body mass index (BMI), 36
Botvin, G. J., 86
brief therapy, 42–43
Bush, R., 113

C
cannabidiol (CBD), 10
Canseco, J., 119–120
cardiovascular effects of AAS, 137–138
case management in treatment, 84
Center for Substance Abuse Treatment (CSAT), 128
central nervous system (CNS) depressants, 3
challenges
  mental game, 57–58
  of trans athletes, 62–65
  physical, 58–59
  technological in sports industry, 65–69
Chang, S., 138
Chauvin, D., 39
Chirico, A., 120
client education in treatment, 84
clinician empathy, 89
Coakley, J., 113
cognitive behavior therapy (CBT), 41–42, 89
cognitive effects of AAS, 138–139
cognitivism theory, 32–33
college athletes, 5–6, 9–17, 59–60. *See also* athlete(s)
  community, 15–16
  cultural factors, 13–14
  drug use among, 73–78
  environmental differences, 14
  family, 15–16
  fans, 15–16
  pain relievers, 12–13
  reasons for using drugs, 12–16

stress reduction, 15
substance use, 82
victims, 14–15
collegiate sports, doping in, 106–113
Comeaux, E., 60
community, 15–16
    college athletes, 15–16
    professional athletes, 24
comorbidity, 127
competitive sports, 51
consultation with other professionals, 85
continued competitiveness, 61–62
Controlled Substances Act (CSA), 9, 11
controlled substances chart, 9
co-occurring disorders, 95–98
Cooley, C. H., 29–30
Corr, C. A., 44
Cottler, L. B., 5, 22
counseling
    addiction, 132–133
    for athlete(s), 98–99, 128–129
    in treatment, 84
COVID-19, 57–59
Creado, S., 5–6
The Criminal Man (Lombroso), 35
crisis intervention in treatment, 84
critical race theory (CRT), 38–39
critical theories, 36–39
cryptocurrency, 66
crypto-wagering sites, 67–68
cultural factors, 13–14
    college athletes, 13–14
    professional athletes, 21–22
cultural lag theory, 28
culture, 75–76

D

Dandoy, C., 106
Darwin's Athletes: How Sport Has Damaged Black America and Preserved the Myth of Race (Hoberman), 53
Darwin's theory, 35
Davies, S., 64
dealing with sports ethics, 102–115
death/dying model, 44–45
Delgado, R., 38
denial, 45
depression, 45, 96
de Shazer, S., 42
developing discrepancies, 42, 89
Dhillon, M., 104
Diagnostic and Statistical Manual of Mental Disorders (DSM-5), 2
DiClemente, C., 41
Dimmock, R., 102

disease model of addiction, 40–41
Doe, J., 132
doping, 21, 97, 106–113
Douglass, F., 37
Drug Enforcement Administration (DEA), 9–10
drugs misuse by athletes, 81–91
    addiction treatment for student athletes, 83–86
    federal laws, 90–91
    intervention strategies, 88–90
    policies, 86–87
    politics, 86–87
    prevention, 86–87
    signs and symptoms, 87–88
drug use
    among collegiate athletes, 73–78
    by sport subculture, 119–122
    prevalence of, 5–6
dual diagnosis, 127
Dworkin, A., 37

E

eating and exercise disorders, 96–97
Elliott, K., 75
empathy, 42
encourage self-efficacy, 89–90
environmental differences, 14
Erikson, E., 32
ethics in sports, 101–115
    academic integrity, 105–106
    dealing with, 102–115
    described, 101–102
    doping in collegiate sports, 106–113
    nanosensors, 113–115
    PEDs, 113
    recruitment and punishment, 103–105
exercise disorders and eating, 96–97

F

family, 15–16
    college athletes, 15–16
    professional athletes, 23–24
Family Educational Rights and Privacy Act (FERPA), 105
fans
    college athletes, 15–16
    professional athletes, 24–25
federal laws, 90–91
Felfe, C., 126
feminist theory, 36–37
fertility, 138
Fisher, A., 102
Food and Drug Administration (FDA), 9
Ford, J. L., 112–113
four stages of addiction model, 40

Freeman, A., 38
Freud, S., 31–32

G
Gallucci, A. R., 5
Ganim, S., 106
gap in social work education, 125–134
    counsel athletes, 128–129
        gaps in addiction counseling, 132–133
        historical thoughts between disciplines, 127–128
        levels of treatment, 130–132
gaps in addiction counseling, 132–133
Gayles, J. G., 75–76
gender, 36–37, 63–64
generalized anxiety disorder (GAD), 96
Gereige, R. S., 106
Gill, E. L., 125
González, J. M. R., 14, 119
Graupensperger, S. A., 77–78
Griffin, K. W., 86
Grobman, A., 125
Guha, N., 4

H
Harbaugh, J., 104
harm reduction model, 43–44
Harper, B., 17, 63
Hauger, L. E., 139
Hawryluk, M., 10
Health Insurance Portability and Accountability Act (HIPAA), 90
Heim, D., 77
Hicks, T., 45
Hirschi, T., 30
HIV/AIDS, 43
Hoberman, J. M., 53
Hollingsworth, J., 64
Holmes, K., 64
Horwitz, H., 138
Hughes, R., 113
hypnotics, 87

I
Ignatow, G., 45
injuries, 95–99
    co-occurring disorders, 95–98
    counseling for athletes, 98–99
International Journal of Sport and Exercise Psychology, 54
intervention strategies, 88–90

J
Jayakumar, U. M., 60
Jellinek, E. M., 40

Jensen, A., 36
Johnson & Johnson/Janssen COVID-19 Vaccine, 59
Juiced (Canseco), 119–120

K
Kant, I, 101
Karst, A., 10
Kissinger, D. B., 59
Kohlberg, L., 33–34, 43
Kübler-Ross, E., 44–45

L
Lal, R., 88
La Vignera, S., 138
Lesser, W. B., 40
Lim, J., 102
Lombroso, C., 35
Lopez, G., 11
Lo, T. W., 89

M
MacKinnon, C., 37
Maclean, S., 39
Maddan, S., 36
Martin, R. J., 5
Mayo Clinic, 87
McGwire, M., 119
McIntosh, P., 37–38
Mead, G. H., 29
Memedovich, K. A., 10
Mendel, J. G., 35
mental game challenges, 57–58
mental health, 1–2, 61–62
    defined, 2
    substance use disorders and, 2–3
Merton, R., 30
Miller, G. A., 127–128
Miller, M. T., 59
Miller, W., 42
Moderna COVID-19 Vaccine, 59
Money, J., 63
Moral Model, 43
moral stages of development, 33–34
Moses, R. A., 76
motivational interviewing (MI), 42, 89
Murray, C., 36

N
nanosensors, 113–115
nanotechnology, 114
National Alliance on Mental Illness (NAMI), 128
National Center for Complementary and Integrative Health (NCCIH), 130

National Collegiate Athletics Association (NCAA), 6, 11, 13, 15, 52, 73–78
    testing, 74–75
National Drug Alliance, 44
Navratilova, M., 64
Nietzsche, F., 115
Nite, C., 76
Nixon, R., 9
nonprescription drugs used, 3–4

O

obsessive-compulsive disorder (OCD), 96
occupational safety and health risks (OSH), 126
Olympics, 121
open-ended questions, 42
operant conditioning, 34
opioids, 22, 87
orientation in treatment, 84
Orsini, M. M., 6
other effects of AAS, 139
oxycontin, 13

P

pain relievers, 12–13
Palmeiro, R., 119
performance-enhancing drugs (PEDs), 120–121
    classes of, 107
    consequences for using, 113
    future challenges, 137–140
    long-term effects of AAS use, 137–139
    sanctions, 108–111
Pfizer BioNTech COVID-19 vaccine, 59
physical challenges, 58–59
physical health, 61–62
Piaget, J., 32–33
Poliakoff, M. B., 106
policies, drugs misuse by athletes, 86–87
politics drugs misuse by athletes, 86–87
Porter, J., 62
prescription drugs, 5, 87
prevention, drugs misuse by athletes, 86–87
Prochaska, J., 41
professional athletes, 6, 21–25. *See also* athlete(s)
    community, 24
    cultural factors, 21–22
    family, 23–24
    fans, 24–25
    victimization, 23
psychiatric effects of AAS, 138–139
psychoanalysis, 31–32
psychological theories, 30–34
psychosexual stages of development, 31
PTSD, 10, 28
pyramiding, 3

R

racism in sports, 52–55
Radcliffe, P., 64
reality principle, 31
Reardon, C. L., 5–6
recruitment and punishment, 103–105
referral in treatment, 84
reflections, 42
regulation, 121
Reimer, D., 63
report and recordkeeping in treatment, 85
reproductive health, 138
Ribeiro, B. G., 4
Robinson, J., 52
Rodriguez, I., 119
rolling with resistance, 42, 89
Rollnick, S., 42
Rubin, L. M., 76
Ruth, B., 51–52

S

Saban, N., 112
Salas-Wright, C. P., 14
Saleeby, D., 40
Sayers, D., 106
Schneider, B., 35
screening in treatment, 84
sedatives, 87
self-efficacy, 42
sexism in sports, 52–55
Sheldon, W., 35–36
signs and symptoms, drugs misuse by athletes, 87–88
Singh, S., 88
six stages of change model, 41
Skinner, B. F., 34
social activities and, 60–61
social anxiety disorder (SAD), 96
social bonding theory, 30
social learning theorists, 30
social work education. *See* gap in social work education
sociological theories, 29–30
sports industry. *See also* ethics in sports
    technological challenges in, 65–69
stacking, 3
Stahl, S., 64
Stambulova, N. B., 58
Stanton, E. C., 37
Stenfancic, J., 38
stimulants, 4, 87
strength-based perspective, 40
stress reduction, 15
student athletes, 83–86
subculture, 76–77, 119–122

substance abuse
  in athletes, 1–2
  counselors, 85, 128
  data, 76
  disorders, 90
Substance Abuse and Mental Health Services Administration (SAMHSA), 128
substance use disorders, 2–3, 97
success or lack of success, 61
summaries, 42
Sutherland, E., 30
symbolic interactionism, 29–30
symbolic interaction theory, 29–30

T

Tatum, J., 59
Technical Assistance Publication Series (TAP), 128
technological challenges in sports industry, 65–69
theories of heredity, 35
theory, defined, 28
theory of body type, 35–36
therapeutic interventions, 39–45
Title 42 of the Code of Federal Regulations Part 2 (42 CFR Part 2), 90–91
Title IX, 64
Toomey, R. B., 64
trans athletes, 62–65
treatment
  addiction, 83–86
  assessment in, 84
  client education in, 84
  counseling in, 84
  crisis intervention in, 84
  intake in, 84
  levels of, 130–132
  orientation in, 84
  plan, 84, 131–132
  report and recordkeeping in, 85
  screening in, 84
Turner, K., 45

U

United States Anti-Doping Agency (USADA), 111–113, 115

V

Vaughn, M. G., 14
victimization, 23
victims, 14–15
Villa, L., 12–13
Vygotsky, L., 32

W

Weaver, E. D. V., 14
Weber, W. S., 119
well-being therapy (WBT), 98
White privilege, 37–38
Wickert, C., 35
women in sports, 52
World Anti-Doping Agency (WADA), 3–4, 11, 111, 115
Wunsch, G., 39

Z

Zhang, A., 66, 106
Zhou, J., 77
Zucker, L., 45

www.ingramcontent.com/pod-product-compliance
Lightning Source LLC
LaVergne TN
LVHW080314260326
834688LV00038B/1108